Balloon pulmonary angioplasty
in patients with CTEPH

Francesco Saia
Nazzareno Galiè · Hiromi Matsubara
Editors

Balloon pulmonary angioplasty in patients with CTEPH

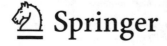

Editors
Francesco Saia
Cardiology Unit, Cardio-Thoracic-
Vascular Department
IRCCS University Hospital of Bologna
Policlinico S.Orsola
Bologna, Italy

Nazzareno Galiè
Cardiology Unit, Cardio-Thoracic-
Vascular Department
IRCCS University Hospital of Bologna
Policlinico S.Orsola
Bologna, Italy

Hiromi Matsubara
Department of Cardiology
National Hospital Organization
Okayama Medical Center
Okayama, Japan

ISBN 978-3-030-95999-9   ISBN 978-3-030-95997-5   (eBook)
https://doi.org/10.1007/978-3-030-95997-5

This Springer imprint is published by the registered company Springer Nature Switzerland AG
The registered company address is: Gewerbestrasse 11, 6330 Cham, Switzerland

Foreword

It was back in the 1980s when studying hemodynamics of patients with chronic lung diseases in Italy we came across a patient with severe pulmonary hypertension, which was difficult to explain by his rather mild COPD. Despite the lack of history of acute pulmonary embolism, his lung scintigraphy showed multiple and large perfusion defects. CT was still to be invented, while standard pulmonary angiography was considered contraindicated in the presence of severe pulmonary hypertension.

Some years later, I realized that this was probably the first patient with chronic thromboembolic pulmonary hypertension (CTEPH) which I have seen. I discovered this while reading an early report from the UC San Diego about surgical treatment of such cases. Frankly, I could not believe that such treatment could be successful. How could you possibly remove large surfaces of intima from pulmonary arterial bed leaving medial layer exposed to blood flow without causing immediate and detrimental thrombosis? Not having the possibility to adequately anticoagulate or thrombolyse the patient with still wide-open sternotomy …? Yet, surgeons performing those ultra-difficult interventions were telling the truth. We owe them many saved patients' lives and their restored happiness.

However, the same surgeons inadvertently delayed the development of another important therapeutic option in CTEPH—percutaneous transcatheter interventions. They had good reasons to discourage interventionists having seen how firm and extensive fibrotic post-thrombotic deposits they needed to tediously remove during pulmonary endarterectomy (PEA) from many pulmonary arterial branches—large and small—to achieve hemodynamic success. This seemed not feasible with any other method than endarterectomy.

Therefore, even though the first reported attempt to perform balloon pulmonary angioplasty (BPA) to treat CTEPH coming from the Netherlands in 1988 was successful, and the first series from the USA published in 2001 was promising, nothing really moved in this direction in countries where PEA surgery blossomed.

How long we would still need to wait if not for our Japanese colleagues, who leapt forward? In relatively short time, they were ready to host the scientific delegation of the most eminent world CTEPH experts and show them what can be achieved with BPA. This great contribution to clinical medicine is reflected by the strong presence of Japanese colleagues among the authors who contributed to this monograph—the first international monograph on all aspects of BPA as a treatment option for CTEPH.

As with all inventions in medicine, new ideas are important, but only if translated into clinically useful implementations which can spread globally. This book will certainly help to disseminate the knowledge about BPA but should also remind us about pioneers and promoters—including the editors of this monograph—who keep trying to define the optimal place for BPA in the CTEPH treatment algorithm in order to provide the greatest benefit to our patients.

Adam Torbicki
Department of Pulmonary Circulation, Thromboembolic
Diseases and Cardiology, Center for Postgraduate Medical Education
Otwock, Poland

Contents

Epidemiology and Pathophysiology of Chronic Thromboembolic Pulmonary Hypertension

Aleksander Kempny, Andrew Constantine, and Colm McCabe

1.1 Epidemiology of Chronic Thromboembolic Pulmonary Hypertension

Chronic thromboembolic pulmonary hypertension (CTEPH), classified as group 4 pulmonary hypertension (PH) in international guidelines, is a progressive disease of obstructive pulmonary arterial remodelling, usually identified as a result of single or multiple episodes of venous thromboembolism (VTE) [1]. Indeed, three-quarters of CTEPH patients report a history of acute pulmonary embolism (PE), with a history of more than one episode of venous thromboembolism (VTE) in 34% [2]. By comparison, a minority of patients do not have a documented history of VTE at presentation. The median age at diagnosis is 63 years with an equal male:female ratio. Paediatric cases are rare [2].

Epidemiological investigation of CTEPH generally accounts for two routes of disease development: firstly, assessment of the cumulative incidence of the disease following an acute PE diagnosis, and secondly, estimation of population prevalence based on national PH registries that include CTEPH patients.

1.2 Risk of Developing CTEPH Following Acute Pulmonary Embolism

Reported incidence of CTEPH following acute PE has varied considerably according to the study population, ranging widely from 0.1 to 11.8% [3–15]. This variability reflects differences between studies in patient selection, CTEPH diagnostic strategies and other methodological differences (Table 1.1). A major limitation in many historical studies is the failure to confirm the diagnosis of PH at right-heart catheterisation in line with diagnostic guidelines. In a meta-analysis of studies employing right-heart catheterisation, the pooled incidence of CTEPH was 0.56% (95% confidence interval, CI 0.1–1.0%) in all comers and 3.2% (95% CI 2–4.4%) in PE survivors [7]. Even amongst these studies, however, there were significant differences in methods employed to screen patients for PH and then

A. Kempny (✉)
Adult Congenital Heart Centre and Centre for Pulmonary Hypertension, Royal Brompton Hospital, Royal Brompton & Harefield Hospitals, Guy's and St Thomas' NHS Foundation Trust, London, UK
e-mail: a.kempny@rbht.nhs.uk

A. Constantine · C. McCabe
Adult Congenital Heart Centre and Centre for Pulmonary Hypertension, Royal Brompton Hospital, Royal Brompton & Harefield Hospitals, Guy's and St Thomas' NHS Foundation Trust, London, UK

National Heart & Lung Institute, Imperial College London, London, UK
e-mail: a.constantine19@imperial.ac.uk;
c.mccabe2@rbht.nhs.uk

© Springer Nature Switzerland AG 2022
F. Saia et al. (eds.), *Balloon pulmonary angioplasty in patients with CTEPH*,
https://doi.org/10.1007/978-3-030-95997-5_1

Table 1.1 Reasons for variability in reported incidence of CTEPH

Patient selection criteria	• Symptomatic PE cases
	• Exclusion of patient groups:
	  – Comorbidities associated with PH (e.g. malignancy, pulmonary disease, left-heart disease)
	  – Past history of PE
	  – Pre-existing dyspnoea
	• Survival to study inclusion

Criteria for CTEPH diagnosis	• echocardiographic screening • definitive diagnostic testing, e.g. by right-heart catheterisation in a subset or not used
Other methodological differences	• cumulative incidence calculated for different length follow-up • intra-study differences in follow-up period between patients • inter-operator variability for estimation of pulmonary artery pressure on echocardiography • different anticoagulation treatment strategies for PE • handling of patients who died between index PE and study inclusion (possibility of undiagnosed PE)

Table 1.2 Putative risk factors and predisposing medical conditions for CTEPH. Modified from [16]

Factors related to the acute PE event	Associated chronic diseases and conditions
Previous VTE	Family history of VTE
High thrombus burden[a]	Congestive heart failure
Echocardiographic signs of pulmonary hypertension/ RV dysfunction at PE diagnosis	Previous splenectomy
CTPA findings suggestive of pre-existing CTEPH	Inflammatory bowel disease
	Chronic deep-seated infection (osteomyelitis, pacemaker wires, indwelling IV lines)
	History of malignancy
	Ventriculo-atrial shunts
	Chronic thyroid replacement therapy
	Non-O blood group

[a] Large pulmonary arterial thrombi on CTPA or large perfusion defect on lung scintigraphy. *CTEPH* chronic thromboembolic pulmonary hypertension, *CTPA* computed tomography pulmonary angiography, *PE* pulmonary embolism, *RV* right ventricle, *VTE* venous thromboembolism.

select for right-heart catheterisation. In some studies, all patients underwent initial echocardiographic screening, whereas in other studies investigations were only initiated in symptomatic patients. Additionally, the lack of investigations prior to a PE diagnosis in all studies raises the additional challenge of differentiating between incident CTEPH following an acute PE, previously unrecognised CTEPH misclassified at presentation and subacute PE in pre-existing CTEPH.

Within the constraints of these technical limitations, however, the following conclusions can be drawn from the literature:

• CTEPH is unlikely to be diagnosed in asymptomatic patients post-PE.
• The vast majority of CTEPH diagnoses post-PE are made within 2 years of diagnosis of the index PE.
• Risk factors for CTEPH following acute PE include recurrent VTE and unprovoked PE [4, 7].

The low incidence of CTEPH in unselected patients following PE led to the 2019 ESC Guidelines for the diagnosis and management of acute PE to recommend screening for CTEPH only in the presence of risk factors (Table 1.2) or dyspnoea and/or functional limitation at 3–6 months following an index event [16].

Epidemiological association between the development of CTEPH and clinical features at the PE presentation includes a more severe index event, as evidenced by a larger perfusion defect on lung scintigraphy [4] or a composite measure of hypotension at PE diagnosis, patient immobilisation or biochemical evidence of myocardial enzyme leak [9, 17]. Studies are conflicting regarding older age at diagnosis as a risk factor [10, 15], with one study identifying older age at diagnosis as a risk factor on multivariate analysis [10]. In studies where patients were not excluded based on comorbidities, a coexistent diagnosis of malignancy, coronary artery disease or chronic obstructive pulmonary disease is commonly encountered.

1.3 Other Clinical Associations of CTEPH

The shortfall in patients where no antecedent VTE can be identified is approximately 30% and, in general, prothrombotic states are not consistently observed in CTEPH. Although prior asymptomatic VTE is recognised [18], marked differences in risk profiles exist between patients with CTEPH and those with isolated VTE indicating that additional unknown factors may be important (Table 1.2).

Further clinical risk factors which have emerged from registry data include history of splenectomy, congestive cardiac failure, family history of VTE, inflammatory bowel disease, infection of indwelling intravenous lines or pacemaker wires, ventriculo-atrial shunts and chronic osteomyelitis [2, 19, 20]. Chronic thyroid replacement therapy and a history of malignancy are more novel risk factors (OR 6.10 and 3.76, respectively) along with chronic Staphylococcal sepsis [21]. CTEPH development also appears more commonly in non-group O compared to group O blood (OR 2.09, 95% CI 1.12–3.94) [19].

1.4 Prognosis Following CTEPH Diagnosis

Patients with CTEPH have the highest survival of all PH groups. This is despite the significant challenge, even in contemporary practice, of a timely diagnosis as evidenced by a median delay to diagnosis of 14 months in the European CTEPH registry [2]. A major component of this success is the transformative, and often curative, value of the surgical management of CTEPH by pulmonary endarterectomy. The UK pulmonary hypertension audit, spanning from 2009 to 2019 at the time of the data presented, illustrates the difference in outcomes between operated and unoperated patients. Of 1237 operated CTEPH patients, the 1- and 5-year survival rates were 95% and 85%, respectively. By comparison, 1583 patients with unoperated CTEPH had a 1- and 5-year survival rates of 86% and 54% [22]. Hence, at present, surgical management is indicated in patients

with disease for which surgery is technically feasible, e.g. more proximal disease adjudicated under current ESC guidelines [1]. Nonetheless, pulmonary endarterectomy is not feasible in all patients, with one-quarter to one-third of cases having distal or microvascular thrombi not amenable to surgery [2]. Furthermore, persistent disease following pulmonary endarterectomy is not uncommon, present in one-half of patients following pulmonary endarterectomy (PEA). This has formed the basis of alternative therapies, including balloon pulmonary angioplasty.

1.5 Pathophysiology of Chronic Thromboembolic Pulmonary Hypertension

The pathological feature of CTEPH is of a progressive fibrotic pulmonary vascular obstruction with organised thrombus, which untreated leads to right ventricular failure. As outlined above, increasing evidence suggests disease development following single or multiple episodes of acute PE; however, where CTEPH is diagnosed outside of this context, other clinical risk factors may predominate. Critical to the disease progression in CTEPH and development of contractile dysfunction of the right ventricle (RV), proximal organised thrombus in main, lobar and segmental territories is accompanied by pathological remodelling in the distal pulmonary vasculature akin to that seen in pulmonary arterial hypertension (PAH). Hypothesised to evolve from overperfusion of unobstructed lung segments, distal vascular remodelling in CTEPH has led to a 'dual compartment' disease model, enhancing our understanding of CTEPH pathobiology and development of treatment strategies [23]. More recently, distal vascular involvement has been shown to serve an important role in disease prognostication for patients undergoing PEA [24]. CTEPH represents a physiological extreme of pulmonary vascular obstruction following acute PE and this contrasts with the more recently coined condition, chronic thromboembolic disease (CTED), where resting PH in response to chronic thrombotic obstruction is not evident.

1.6 Abnormal Thrombus Resolution

A majority consensus on the aetiology of CTEPH has emerged predicated on a theory of disordered thrombus resolution following acute VTE/PE [2]. Integral to this concept is the degradation and removal of acute large-vessel thrombi in the non-diseased state and whether individuals predisposed to CTEPH respond differently following acute PE. Experimental evidence of abnormal thrombus resolution first emerged in animal models where pharmacological inhibition of fibrinolysis potentiated the development of organised pulmonary thrombus [25]. This raised suspicion that patients with CTEPH may harbour a fibrinolytic genetic defect; indeed, in vitro dysfibrinogenaemia identified in the peripheral blood of CTEPH patients suggests that this population may harbour fibrin variants with enhanced resistance to lysis [26].

Under normal circumstances, acute thrombus degradation involves a complex process of adaptive thrombus remodelling, neovascularisation and recanalisation of the pulmonary artery wall. Recruitment and margination of monocytes and neutrophils enhance thrombus clearance by recruitment of inflammatory mediators which upregulate growth factor expression. These include vascular endothelial growth factor (VEGF) known to enhance tissue factor mRNA and protein levels on endothelial cells [27], transforming growth factor-beta (TGF-β), fibroblastic growth factor (FGF), proteases (matrix metallopeptidases/urokinase-type plasminogen activator) and chemoattractants, all of which accelerate the organisation and resolution of venous thrombi [28].

In CTEPH, deregulation of monocyte recruitment has been shown to be detrimental to this process with significant elevation in interleukin (IL)-10, monocyte chemotactic protein-1 and matrix metallopeptidase (MMP)-9 found in peripheral blood of patients with CTEPH [29, 30]. Surgical PEA specimens in CTEPH demonstrate abundant macrophages, lymphocytes and neutrophils supporting an inflammatory substrate in the non-resolution of thrombus. In contrast to acute PE thrombus, histological examination of PEA specimens demonstrates a fibrotic meshwork of collagen, elastin and inflammatory cells. However, histological specimens also highlight a paucity of vessel penetration within obstructive material suggesting that deficient angiogenesis may be a driver of occlusive vascular remodelling and/or inadequate recanalisation of thrombotic material. These findings are supported by increased levels of platelet factor 4, collagen type I and C-X-C motif chemokine ligand 10 (CXCL10), angiostatic factors which are associated with decreased proliferation and angiogenesis [31]. Despite well-conducted descriptive analyses, the individual contributions of these factors to cellular remodelling, inflammation and neovascularisation, which ultimately culminate in delayed thrombus resolution, remain subject to debate.

1.7 Further Haematological Abnormalities

Platelets play a key role in coagulation and haemostasis, but their role in the development of CTEPH is less clear. Patients with CTEPH display decreased platelet counts, higher mean platelet volume and differences in platelet aggregation in support of a prothrombotic state. Platelet activation defined by increased P-selectin and glycoprotein IIb/IIIa levels is also enhanced in CTEPH patients compared to patients with PAH and controls although the impact of having PH in this context is not well defined. Surgical PEA specimens demonstrate reduced expression of platelet endothelial cell adhesion molecule-1 (PECAM-1), a glycoprotein involved in leucocyte transmigration, in comparison to non-thrombosed vessels suggesting that PECAM-1 deficiency may be important to thrombus degradation.

Plasmatic risk factors have been the subject of detailed investigation with traditional prothrombotic factors explaining less than 10% of reported CTEPH cases. In particular, deficiency in antithrombin, protein C or protein S, all known to predispose to recurrent VTE, share no association with CTEPH. Similarly, mutation in factor V R506Q (factor V Leiden) appears to be unrelated to CTEPH development. In contrast, high titres of antiphospholipid antibodies have been demonstrated in patients with CTEPH as well as increased factor VIII and von Willebrand factor antigen levels (VWF:Ag) [19, 32–34]. The presence of a lupus anticoagulant, strongly associated with recurrent VTE, also accounts for a minority of cases [35].

1.8 Genetic Differences in CTEPH Patients

Rare genetic variants within the fibrinogen gene have been associated with relative resistance to plasminogen-mediated fibrinolysis [36]. This was demonstrated by an over-represented fibrinogen A alpha-chain Thr312Ala polymorphism in a small CTEPH cohort [37]. A larger study in 2013 confirmed this finding where patients with a higher allele frequency for this polymorphism were found to harbour a higher resistance to fibrinolysis [38]. Two further candidate polymorphisms in the endoglin and MAPK 10 genes emerged as risk factors for CTEPH in a Chinese population [39]. However, none of these studies confirmed downstream in vivo effects of the identified polymorphisms. Mutations in seven genes related to forms of PH other than CTEPH (BMPR2, ENG, SMAD9, CAV1, KCNK3, ACVRL1 and CBLN2) have also been studied and in total, 25 non-synonymous mutations amongst these genes were detected in CTEPH patients with the majority predicted to harbour deleterious effects. A further underpowered genome-wide association study demonstrated association between HLA loci B*5201 and DPB1*0202 in patients with CTEPH [40], although no downstream protein target has been identified. Studies investigating BMPR2 mutations in CTEPH patients in Europe have failed to detect any known mutations [41, 42]. This suggests that larger patient cohorts are required to fully elucidate the frequency of the described mutations in CTEPH patients, as well as uncover regional variation in the mutation frequency [43].

Human gene expression studies in CTEPH are even more rare. Comparing CTEPH thrombi and native pulmonary arterial tissue samples obtained at surgery, abnormal regulation of pathways involved with proliferation and endothelial function has been identified [44]. Gu et al. performed a complementary DNA (cDNA) array analysis of pulmonary artery endothelial cells obtained from 5 CTEPH patients and controls finding 1614 genes differentially expressed between the two groups [45]. Genetic expression differed predominantly in pathways involving cell proliferation, signal transduction and cytokine pathways, in particular the mitogen-activated protein kinase (MAPK) pathway and phosphoinositide 3-kinase (PI3K) pathway. In the post-translational domain, mutations have also been identified in untranslated genomic regions in CTEPH which is important given the potential for post-transcriptional regulation by microRNAs. MicroRNAs are short (~22 nucleotides) non-coding RNAs, which, through sequence-specific interaction with target sites in the 3′ untranslated region (3′UTR) of messenger RNAs (mRNA), moderate the levels of mRNA available for translation. Chen et al. first identified association between microRNAs and CTEPH identifying miR-759 involvement in the degradation of fibrinogen mRNA in the liver [46]. Two further microRNAs, miR-22 and let-7b, are downregulated in peripheral blood in CTEPH patients with let-7b implicated in TGF-β and ET-1 expression [47]. MicroRNA network analysis remains at an early stage, however, and further studies of functional effects of microRNAs implicated in vascular remodelling will further advance this field.

1.9 Small-Vessel Disease in CTEPH

In addition to proximal thrombotic obstructive lesions, post-mortem studies in CTEPH were first to identify the presence of small-vessel lesions similar to those present in idiopathic PAH [48]. Pathological changes were characterised by vessel intimal thickening and fibrosis, remodelled pulmonary resistive vessels and plexiform lesions. Clinically, small-vessel disease is suspected when the burden of larger vessel obstruction or narrowing fails to account for the degree of elevation in pulmonary vascular resistance. Small-vessel disease may arise due to higher small-vessel wall shear stress given reciprocal increases in flow in response to obstructed lung segments. However, characteristic vascular remodelling has also been identified within vessels *downstream* of fibrotic occlusions. More contemporary pathological examination in CTEPH has highlighted prominent large anastomoses between the systemic and pulmonary arterial circulation consisting of hypertrophied bronchial vessels [49]. The authors speculated as to whether pre-existing vascular anastomoses may be enlarged by an increased pressure gradient between bronchial and pulmonary vessels which more distally may be patent. Finally, pathological examination of non-obstructed and obstructed lung segments in CTEPH undertaken following PEA has demonstrated that partitioning of pulmonary vascular resistance may predict the development of post-operative PH through evaluation of the pulmonary artery occlusion waveform [24]. This suggests the potentially intriguing possibility to investigate for the presence or absence of small-vessel disease in CTED in the small numbers who undergo surgery in an attempt to better understand the evolution of this condition.

1.10   Molecular Pathways

As in PAH, the nitric oxide pathway has been implicated in the pathogenesis of CTEPH-associated small-vessel remodelling given reduced nitric oxide (NO) synthase activity and reduced endogenous NO levels. Clinical improvements in CTEPH patients in response to Riociguat, a soluble guanylate cyclase stimulator which augments the NO-cGMP axis, suggest significant contribution from this pathway to target small-vessel involvement in CTEPH [50, 51]. Increased levels of endothelin-1 (ET-1) and angiopoietin-1 in CTEPH support a further substrate for the enhancement of smooth muscle pro-

liferation [52, 53]. Although the efficacy of endothelin receptor antagonists as monotherapy may be less robust, there remains a clinical appetite for their continued use in CTEPH [54].

1.11   Right Ventricular Dysfunction in CTEPH

Raised afterload arising from thrombotic obstruction in CTEPH increases the mechanical load on the RV. RV hypertrophy is a physiological response to increased afterload which maintains wall stress within normal limits and so improves mechanical pump efficiency. Changes in RV contractile performance have been explored in both patients with CTEPH and patients with CTED in whom pulmonary artery pressures are maintained closer to normal limits despite a large burden of chronic thrombotic obstruction in the main pulmonary arteries. Using conductance catheterisation, differences between patients with CTEPH, CTED and controls were observed by pressure-volume loop morphology, most notably during RV systolic ejection [55]. In patients with CTED, these changes resulted from the elevated RV afterload that develops independent of PH and predisposes to characteristic changes during exercise adaptation of the pulmonary circulation represented during cardiopulmonary exercise testing [56]. A further large animal study using a pulmonary artery banding model suggested that ventriculo-arterial coupling, again measured by pressure-volume catheterisation, may be used to define an 'optimal threshold' for RV mechanical efficiency either side of which cardiac output and stroke work begin to decrease (Fig. 1.1) [57]. This identified an Ees/Ea value of 0.68 ± 0.23 suggesting that patients with CTED may harbour occult RV dysfunction that cannot be identified by more routine methods of evaluation.

Further insight into the capacity of the RV to reverse remodel may be gleaned from post-surgical interrogation of RV function and from assessment in patients following balloon pulmonary angioplasty (BPA). Surgical treatment of CTEPH alleviates systolic RV wall stress which appears key to the re-establishment of contractile synchrony

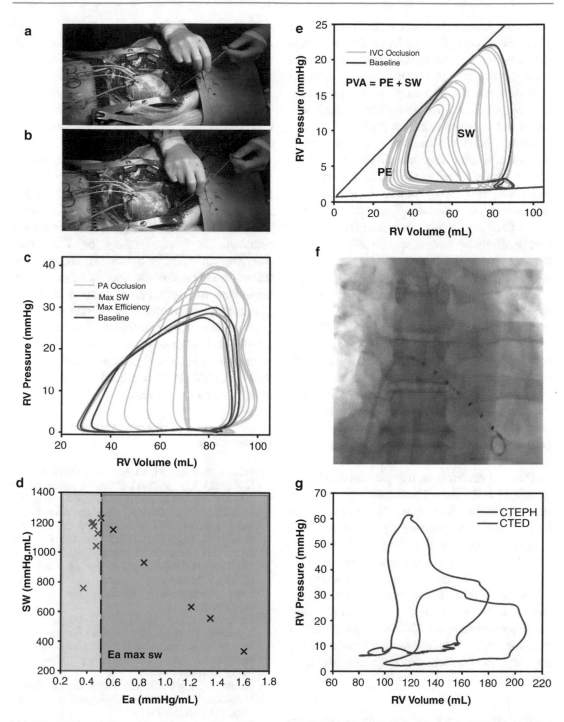

Fig. 1.1 (**a**) Animal model porcine heart instrumented with conductance catheter; (**b**) with PA snare partially occluded to increase RV afterload; (**c**) RV PV loops recorded during the PA snare. PV loops are highlighted at baseline (blue), maximal efficiency (green) and maximal SW (red). (**d**) SW-Ea RV PV loop relationship during the PA snare, (green) RV energetic reserve, (red) RV failure. (**e**) RV PV loops recorded during an IVC occlusion. PV loops are highlighted at baseline (blue). SW is highlighted as the area contained within the baseline RV PV loop. PE is the area within the Ees and EDPVR pressure volume relationships. (**f**) Fluoroscopic image of conductance catheter located in the RV during the clinical study; (**g**) typical RV PV loop morphology recorded for patients with CTED (blue) or CTEPH (red) [57]

between right and left ventricles [58]. Improvements in RV function following BPA are less well studied; however a recent meta-analysis supports the use of imaging as a valid modality to follow patients after BPA and, from a total of 14 included studies, showed significant improvements in haemodynamic and imaging parameters [59].

Metabolic RV dysfunction is an evolving topic but remains relatively unexplored in CTEPH until recently. Dysfunctional RV hypertrophic tissue has been demonstrated to metabolically switch energy substrates from mitochondria-based fatty acid oxidation to less efficient glycolysis. Surgical treatment with PEA confirms the capacity of the RV to reverse remodel, a pathway which represents an exciting route to interrogate changes in RV metabolic perturbation secondary to increased afterload. Swietlik et al. explored RV metabolic changes in CTEPH recently using an invasive trans-RV and transpulmonary approach to measure metabolite gradients in CTEPH [60]. They demonstrated metabolites relevant to CTEPH pathobiology and metabolic gradients which are associated with clinical measures of disease severity, informing potentially novel mechanisms of RV and pulmonary vascular adaptation. Simmoneau et al. in their recent review raise the question of whether an unloaded RV should be considered 'preconditioned' and therefore be expected to better sustain a potential increase in afterload [61]. Speculation that irreversible damage from sustained increase in afterload may confer a 'point of no return' for the RV somewhere along the sequence of events induced by CTEPH will require better understanding of the longitudinal consequences of both CTED and acute PE on RV function, which, due to evolving definitions and severity classifications, may not necessarily carry similar physiological effects [62].

1.12 Conclusion

The diagnostic criteria for CTEPH have remained consistent since their formal definition by Moser in 1990. Since this time, advances in our understanding of its pathophysiology, in particular the role of acute PE, infection, inflammation and haematological abnormalities, have placed the present-day PH community in a far stronger position to identify and treat CTEPH earlier. Future identification of genetic and molecular signatures of CTEPH is also more likely given wider application of screening in larger populations. The spectrum of CTEPH management now includes not only patients with confirmed PH but also an evolving patient group who do not meet haemodynamic cut-offs for PH at rest yet harbour pulmonary thrombosis-related exercise limitation. The biology of this patient group remains largely unknown; however, it may be the 'dual-compartment' CTEPH model that requires further refinement as maladaptation of the pulmonary circulation to acute PE is better understood. Therapeutic intervention beyond routine anticoagulation aimed at preventing the development of CTEPH and progression to RV failure represents an exciting goal, although identification of relevant biological targets in predisposed individuals remains elusive at present.

References

1. Galiè N, Humbert M, Vachiery J-L, Gibbs S, Lang I, Torbicki A, et al. 2015 ESC/ERS guidelines for the diagnosis and treatment of pulmonary hypertension: the joint task force for the diagnosis and treatment of pulmonary hypertension of the European Society of Cardiology (ESC) and the European Respiratory Society (ERS): endorsed by: Association for European Paediatric and Congenital Cardiology (AEPC), International Society for Heart and Lung Transplantation (ISHLT). Eur Heart J. 2015;37(1):67–119.
2. Pepke-Zaba J, Delcroix M, Lang I, Mayer E, Jansa P, Ambroz D, et al. Chronic thromboembolic pulmonary hypertension (CTEPH): results from an international prospective registry. Circulation. 2011;124(18):1973–81.
3. Fedullo PF, Auger WR, Kerr KM, Rubin LJ. Chronic thromboembolic pulmonary hypertension. N Engl J Med. 2001;345(20):1465–72.
4. Pengo V, Lensing AW, Prins MH, Marchiori A, Davidson BL, Tiozzo F, et al. Incidence of chronic thromboembolic pulmonary hypertension after pulmonary embolism. N Engl J Med. 2004;350(22):2257–64.
5. Klok FA, Zondag W, van Kralingen KW, van Dijk AP, Tamsma JT, Heyning FH, et al. Patient outcomes after acute pulmonary embolism. A pooled survival analy-

sis of different adverse events. Am J Respir Crit Care Med. 2010;181(5):501–6.

6. Golpe R, Pérez-de-Llano LA, Castro-Añón O, Vázquez-Caruncho M, González-Juanatey C, Veres-Racamonde A, et al. Right ventricle dysfunction and pulmonary hypertension in hemodynamically stable pulmonary embolism. Respir Med. 2010;104(9):1370–6.

7. Ende-Verhaar YM, Cannegieter SC, Vonk Noordegraaf A, Delcroix M, Pruszczyk P, Mairuhu ATA, et al. Incidence of chronic thromboembolic pulmonary hypertension after acute pulmonary embolism: a contemporary view of the published literature. Eur Respir J. 2017;49(2):1601792.

8. Miniati M, Monti S, Bottai M, Scoscia E, Bauleo C, Tonelli L, et al. Survival and restoration of pulmonary perfusion in a Long-term follow-up of patients after acute pulmonary embolism. Medicine. 2006;85(5):253 62.

9. Otero R, Oribe M, Ballaz A, Jimenez D, Uresandi F, Nauffal D, et al. Echocardiographic assessment of pulmonary arterial pressure in the follow-up of patients with pulmonary embolism. Thromb Res. 2011;127(4):303–8.

10. Martí D, Gómez V, Escobar C, Wagner C, Zamarro C, Sánchez D, et al. Incidence of symptomatic and asymptomatic chronic thromboembolic pulmonary hypertension. Arch Bronconeumol. 2010;46(12):628–33.

11. Surie S, Gibson NS, Gerdes VEA, Bouma BJ, BLF VES, Buller HR, et al. Active search for chronic thromboembolic pulmonary hypertension does not appear indicated after acute pulmonary embolism. Thromb Res. 2010;125(5):e202–e5.

12. Poli D, Grifoni E, Antonucci E, Arcangeli C, Prisco D, Abbate R, et al. Incidence of recurrent venous thromboembolism and of chronic thromboembolic pulmonary hypertension in patients after a first episode of pulmonary embolism. Thromb Res. 2010;30(3):294–9.

13. Dentali F, Donadini M, Gianni M, Bertolini A, Squizzato A, Venco A, et al. Incidence of chronic pulmonary hypertension in patients with previous pulmonary embolism. Thromb Res. 2009;124(3):256–8.

14. Becattini C, Agnelli G, Pesavento R, Silingardi M, Poggio R, Taliani MR, et al. Incidence of chronic thromboembolic pulmonary hypertension after a first episode of pulmonary embolism. Chest. 2006;130(1):172–5.

15. Ribeiro A, Lindmarker P, Johnsson H, Juhlin-Dannfelt A, Jorfeldt L. Pulmonary embolism: one-year follow-up with echocardiography doppler and five-year survival analysis. Circulation. 1999;99(10):1325–30.

16. Konstantinides SV, Meyer G, Becattini C, Bueno H, Geersing G-J, Harjola V-P, et al. ESC guidelines for the diagnosis and management of acute pulmonary embolism developed in collaboration with the European Respiratory Society (ERS): the task force for the diagnosis and management of acute pulmonary embolism of the European Society of Cardiology (ESC). Eur Heart J. 2019;41(4):543–603.

17. Lankeit M, Kempf T, Dellas C, Cuny M, Tapken H, Peter T, et al. Growth differentiation factor-15 for prognostic assessment of patients with acute pulmonary embolism. Am J Respir Crit Care Med. 2008;177(9):1018–25.

18. Dartevelle P, Fadel E, Mussot S, Chapelier A, Herve P, de Perrot M, et al. Chronic thromboembolic pulmonary hypertension. Eur Respir J. 2004;23(4):637–48.

19. Bonderman D, Wilkens H, Wakounig S, Schafers HJ, Jansa P, Lindner J, et al. Risk factors for chronic thromboembolic pulmonary hypertension. Eur Respir J. 2009;33(2):325–31.

20. Lang IM, Simonneau G, Pepke-Zaba JW, Mayer E, Ambrož D, Blanco I, et al. Factors associated with diagnosis and operability of chronic thromboembolic pulmonary hypertension. A case-control study. Thromb Haemost. 2013;110(1):83–91.

21. Bonderman D, Jakowitsch J, Redwan B, Bergmeister H, Renner MK, Panzenbock H, et al. Role for staphylococci in misguided thrombus resolution of chronic thromboembolic pulmonary hypertension. Arterioscler Thromb Vasc Biol. 2008;28(4):678–84.

22. Digital N (2019) National audit of pulmonary hypertension great Britain, 2018–19. Tenth annual report. https://digital.nhs.uk/data-and-information/publications/statistical/national-pulmonary-hypertension-audit/2019. 24 Oct 2019

23. Kim NH. Group 4 pulmonary hypertension: chronic thromboembolic pulmonary hypertension: epidemiology, pathophysiology, and treatment. Cardiol Clin. 2016;34(3):435–41.

24. Gerges C, Gerges M, Friewald R, Fesler P, Dorfmüller P, Sharma S, et al. Microvascular disease in chronic thromboembolic pulmonary hypertension: hemodynamic phenotyping and Histomorphometric assessment. Circulation. 2020;141(5):376–86.

25. Moser KM, Cantor JP, Olman M, Villespin I, Graif JL, Konopka R, et al. Chronic pulmonary thromboembolism in dogs treated with tranexamic acid. Circulation. 1991;83(4):1371–9.

26. Morris TA, Marsh JJ, Chiles PG, Auger WR, Fedullo PF, Woods VL Jr. Fibrin derived from patients with chronic thromboembolic pulmonary hypertension is resistant to lysis. Am J Respir Crit Care Med. 2006;173(11):1270–5.

27. Mechtcheriakova D, Wlachos A, Holzmuller H, Binder BR, Hofer E. Vascular endothelial cell growth factor-induced tissue factor expression in endothelial cells is mediated by EGR-1. Blood. 1999;93(11):3811–23.

28. Waltham M, Burnand KG, Collins M, McGuinness CL, Singh I, Smith A. Vascular endothelial growth factor enhances venous thrombus recanalisation and organisation. Thromb Haemost. 2003;89(1):169–76.

29. McGuinness CL, Humphries J, Waltham M, Burnand KG, Collins M, Smith A. Recruitment of labelled monocytes by experimental venous thrombi. Thromb Haemost. 2001;85(6):1018–24.

30. Ali T, Humphries J, Burnand K, Sawyer B, Bursill C, Channon K, et al. Monocyte recruitment in venous thrombus resolution. J Vasc Surg. 2006;43(3):601–8.

31. Zabini D, Nagaraj C, Stacher E, Lang IM, Nierlich P, Klepetko W, et al. Angiostatic factors in the pulmonary endarterectomy material from chronic thromboembolic pulmonary hypertension patients cause endothelial dysfunction. PLoS One. 2012;7(8):e43793.

32. Bonderman D, Turecek PL, Jakowitsch J, Weltermann A, Adlbrecht C, Schneider B, et al. High prevalence of elevated clotting factor VIII in chronic thromboembolic pulmonary hypertension. Thromb Haemost. 2003;90(3):372–6.

33. Wolf M, Boyer-Neumann C, Parent F, Eschwege V, Jaillet H, Meyer D, et al. Thrombotic risk factors in pulmonary hypertension. Eur Respir J. 2000;15(2):395–9.

34. Wong CL, Szydlo R, Gibbs S, Laffan M. Hereditary and acquired thrombotic risk factors for chronic thromboembolic pulmonary hypertension. Blood Coagul Fibrinolysis. 2010;21(3):201–6.

35. Auger WR, Permpikul P, Moser KM. Lupus anticoagulant, heparin use, and thrombocytopenia in patients with chronic thromboembolic pulmonary hypertension: a preliminary report. Am J Med. 1995;99(4):392–6.

36. Linenberger ML, Kindelan J, Bennett RL, Reiner AP, Cote HC. Fibrinogen Bellingham: a gamma-chain R275C substitution and a beta-promoter polymorphism in a thrombotic member of an asymptomatic family. Am J Hematol. 2000;64(4):242–50.

37. Suntharalingam J, Goldsmith K, van Marion V, Long L, Treacy CM, Dudbridge F, et al. Fibrinogen Aalpha Thr312Ala polymorphism is associated with chronic thromboembolic pulmonary hypertension. Eur Respir J. 2008;31(4):736–41.

38. Li JF, Lin Y, Yang YH, Gan HL, Liang Y, Liu J, et al. Fibrinogen alpha Thr312Ala polymorphism specifically contributes to chronic thromboembolic pulmonary hypertension by increasing fibrin resistance. PLoS One. 2013;8(7):e69635.

39. Xi Q, Liu Z, Zhao Z, Luo Q, Huang Z. High frequency of pulmonary hypertension-causing gene mutation in Chinese patients with chronic thromboembolic pulmonary hypertension. PLoS One. 2016;11(1):e0147396.

40. Kominami S, Tanabe N, Ota M, Naruse TK, Katsuyama Y, Nakanishi N, et al. HLA-DPB1 and NFKBIL1 may confer the susceptibility to chronic thromboembolic pulmonary hypertension in the absence of deep vein thrombosis. J Hum Genet. 2009;54(2):108–14.

41. Ulrich S, Szamalek-Hoegel J, Hersberger M, Fischler M, Garcia JS, Huber LC, et al. Sequence variants in BMPR2 and genes involved in the serotonin and nitric oxide pathways in idiopathic pulmonary arterial hypertension and chronic thromboembolic pulmonary hypertension: relation to clinical parameters and comparison with left heart disease. Respiration. 2010;79(4):279–87.

42. Suntharalingam J, Machado RD, Sharples LD, Toshner MR, Sheares KK, Hughes RJ, et al. Demographic features, BMPR2 status and outcomes in distal chronic thromboembolic pulmonary hypertension. Thorax. 2007;62(7):617–22.

43. Opitz I, Kirschner MB. Molecular research in chronic thromboembolic pulmonary hypertension. Int J Mol Sci. 2019;20(3)

44. Lang IM, Marsh JJ, Olman MA, Moser KM, Loskutoff DJ, Schleef RR. Expression of type 1 plasminogen activator inhibitor in chronic pulmonary thromboemboli. Circulation. 1994;89(6):2715–21.

45. Gu S, Su P, Yan J, Zhang X, An X, Gao J, et al. Comparison of gene expression profiles and related pathways in chronic thromboembolic pulmonary hypertension. Int J Mol Med. 2014;33(2):277–300.

46. Chen Z, Nakajima T, Tanabe N, Hinohara K, Sakao S, Kasahara Y, et al. Susceptibility to chronic thromboembolic pulmonary hypertension may be conferred by miR-759 via its targeted interaction with polymorphic fibrinogen alpha gene. Hum Genet. 2010;128(4):443–52.

47. Wang L, Guo LJ, Liu J, Wang W, Yuan JX, Zhao L, et al. MicroRNA expression profile of pulmonary artery smooth muscle cells and the effect of let-7d in chronic thromboembolic pulmonary hypertension. Pulm Circ. 2013;3(3):654–64.

48. Moser KM, Bloor CM. Pulmonary vascular lesions occurring in patients with chronic major vessel thromboembolic pulmonary hypertension. Chest. 1993;103(3):685–92.

49. Dorfmuller P, Gunther S, Ghigna MR, Thomas de Montpreville V, Boulate D, Paul JF, et al. Microvascular disease in chronic thromboembolic pulmonary hypertension: a role for pulmonary veins and systemic vasculature. Eur Respir J. 2014;44(5):1275–88.

50. Ghofrani HA, D'Armini AM, Grimminger F, Hoeper MM, Jansa P, Kim NH, et al. Riociguat for the treatment of chronic thromboembolic pulmonary hypertension. N Engl J Med. 2013;369(4):319–29.

51. Simonneau G, D'Armini AM, Ghofrani HA, Grimminger F, Hoeper MM, Jansa P, et al. Riociguat for the treatment of chronic thromboembolic pulmonary hypertension: a long-term extension study (CHEST-2). Eur Respir J. 2015;45(5):1293–302.

52. Southwood M, MacKenzie Ross RV, Kuc RE, Hagan G, Sheares KK, Jenkins DP, et al. Endothelin ETA receptors predominate in chronic thromboembolic pulmonary hypertension. Life Sci. 2016;159:104–10.

53. Hoeper MM, Mayer E, Simonneau G, Rubin LJ. Chronic thromboembolic pulmonary hypertension. Circulation. 2006;113(16):2011–20.

54. Jais X, D'Armini AM, Jansa P, Torbicki A, Delcroix M, Ghofrani HA, et al. Bosentan for treatment of inoperable chronic thromboembolic pulmonary hypertension: BENEFiT (Bosentan effects in iNopErable forms of chronIc thromboembolic pulmonary hypertension), a randomized, placebo-controlled trial. J Am Coll Cardiol. 2008;52(25):2127–34.

55. McCabe C, White PA, Hoole SP, Axell RG, Priest AN, Gopalan D, et al. Right ventricular dysfunction in chronic thromboembolic obstruction of the pulmonary artery: a pressure-volume study using the conductance catheter. J Appl Physiol (1985). 2014;116(4):355–363.
56. McCabe C, Deboeck G, Harvey I, Ross RM, Gopalan D, Screaton N, et al. Inefficient exercise gas exchange identifies pulmonary hypertension in chronic thromboembolic obstruction following pulmonary embolism. Thromb Res. 2013;132(6):659–65.
57. Axell RG, Messer SJ, White PA, McCabe C, Priest A, Statopoulou T, et al. Ventriculo-arterial coupling detects occult RV dysfunction in chronic thromboembolic pulmonary vascular disease. Physiol Rep. 2017;5(7)
58. Mauritz GJ, Vonk-Noordegraaf A, Kind T, Surie S, Kloek JJ, Bresser P, et al. Pulmonary endarterectomy normalizes interventricular dyssynchrony and right ventricular systolic wall stress. J Cardiovasc Magn Reson. 2012;14:5.
59. Karyofyllis P, Demerouti E, Papadopoulou V, Voudris V, Matsubara H. Balloon pulmonary angioplasty as a treatment in chronic thromboembolic pulmonary hypertension: past, present, and future. Curr Treat Options Cardiovasc Med. 2020;22(3):7.
60. Swietlik EM, Ghataorhe P, Zalewska KI, Wharton J, Howard LS, Taboada D, et al. Plasma metabolomics exhibit response to therapy in chronic thromboembolic pulmonary hypertension. Eur Respir J. 2020;2020:15.
61. Simonneau G, Torbicki A, Dorfmuller P, Kim N. The pathophysiology of chronic thromboembolic pulmonary hypertension. Eur Respir Rev. 2017;26:143.
62. McCabe C, Dimopoulos K, Pitcher A, Orchard E, Price LC, Kempny A, et al. Chronic thromboembolic disease following pulmonary embolism: time for a fresh look at old clot. Eur Respir J. 2020;55(4)

Diagnosis of Chronic Thromboembolic Pulmonary Hypertension

Massimiliano Palazzini, Francesco Saia,
Daniele Guarino, Nevio Taglieri,
Alessandra Manes, Nazzareno Galiè,
and Fabio Dardi

Abbreviations

BPA	Balloon pulmonary angioplasty
CTEPH	Chronic thromboembolic pulmonary hypertension
CTPA	Computed tomography pulmonary angiography
HRTC	High-resolution CT
mPAP	Mean pulmonary artery pressure
MRI	Magnetic resonance imaging
PAH	Pulmonary arterial hypertension
PAWP	Pulmonary artery wedge pressure
PE	Pulmonary embolism
PEA	Pulmonary endarterectomy
PH	Pulmonary hypertension
PVOD	Pulmonary veno-occlusive disease
PVR	Pulmonary vascular resistance
RHC	Right-heart catheterisation
V/Q	Ventilation/perfusion lung scan

M. Palazzini (✉) · N. Galiè
Cardiology Unit, Cardio-Thoracic-Vascular
Department, IRCCS University Hospital of
Bologna, Policlinico S. Orsola, Bologna, Italy

Department of Experimental, Diagnostic and
Specialty Medicine (DIMES), Bologna University
Hospital, Bologna, Italy
e-mail: massimiliano.palazzini@unibo.it;
nazzareno.galie@unibo.it

F. Saia · N. Taglieri · A. Manes
Cardiology Unit, Cardio-Thoracic-Vascular
Department, IRCCS University Hospital of Bologna,
Policlinico S. Orsola, Bologna, Italy
e-mail: francesco.saia@unibo.it;
nevio.taglieri@aosp.bo.it; alessandra.manes@unibo.it

D. Guarino · F. Dardi
Department of Experimental, Diagnostic and
Specialty Medicine (DIMES), Bologna University
Hospital, Bologna, Italy
e-mail: daniele.guarino3@unibo.it;
fabio.dardi@aosp.bo.it

2.1 Introduction

Chronic thromboembolic pulmonary hypertension (CTEPH) is classified within group 4 of the clinical classification of pulmonary hypertension (PH) [1], and it is pathologically characterised by the presence of organised thromboembolic material, such as ring-like stenoses, webs/slits and chronic total occlusions (pouch lesions or tapered lesions), and by altered vascular remodelling associated with precapillary PH. The diagnosis of CTEPH is based on findings obtained after at least 3 months of effective anticoagulation in order to discriminate this condition from "subacute" pulmonary embolism. CTEPH is haemodynamically defined by the presence of precapillary PH (mean pulmonary artery pressure (mPAP) ≥ 25 mmHg, pulmonary artery wedge pressure (PAWP) ≤ 15 mmHg, pulmonary vascular resistance (PVR) >3 WU) as assessed by right-heart catheterisation (RHC), together with multiple perfusion defects [1].

© Springer Nature Switzerland AG 2022
F. Saia et al. (eds.), *Balloon pulmonary angioplasty in patients with CTEPH*,
https://doi.org/10.1007/978-3-030-95997-5_2

Being able to diagnose CTEPH is extremely important because it is the only potentially curable form of PH and because of its poor prognosis if left untreated, especially in case of severe PH [2, 3]. Early diagnosis, however, remains challenging in CTEPH, with a median time of 14 months between symptom onset and diagnosis in expert centres [4]. Some patients enter the diagnostic process with unclear symptoms suggestive of PH, while others are suspected to have CTEPH based on their history or risk factors such as recurrent venous thromboembolism, antiphospholipid antibodies and lupus anticoagulant, inflammatory bowel disease, ventriculo-atrial shunt, cardiac pacemaker, a history of splenectomy or thyroid hormone replacement [5]. Patients who are diagnosed with acute pulmonary embolism (PE) but show signs of chronic disease should be explored for CTEPH. Importantly, however, the absence of previous history of acute PE does not exclude CTEPH. Physical examination, standard laboratory tests, chest X-ray, electrocardiogram, echocardiogram and RHC may provide no differential clues between CTEPH and pulmonary arterial hypertension (PAH).

Identifying CTEPH as the cause of PH is an investigative process that combines several high-quality imaging techniques, on the one hand, and assessment of the haemodynamic profile with RHC on the other. The former include ventilation/perfusion (V/Q) lung scan, computed tomography pulmonary angiography (CTPA), high-resolution CT (HRCT), magnetic resonance imaging (MRI) and pulmonary angiography with or without digital subtraction. These diagnostic tools are useful to define the presence, location and distribution of perfusion defects throughout the pulmonary circulation. RHC is just as important to confirm the diagnosis and provides further information on the degree of haemodynamic impairment that can result from perfusion abnormalities. In all cases, the diagnostic workup should be completed by detailed medical history, physical examination and transthoracic echocardiography. Echocardiogram can provide initial clues towards the diagnosis either by documenting an increased estimated systolic pulmonary arterial pressure or by showing signs of right ventricular pressure overload, such as right ventricular hypertrophy and dilation and systolic flattening of the interventricular septum [1]. In some cases, large organised thrombotic clots can also be documented in the main pulmonary artery and its bifurcation by ultrasound technique. Being a quite inexpensive diagnostic tool, echocardiogram should always be performed when suspecting CTEPH, especially when searching for potential causes of heart failure in patients with a previous history of pulmonary embolism [1]. The combination of imaging and functional investigations is mandatory in the diagnostic strategy of CTEPH as it might provide essential information for early establishment of appropriate treatment. In latest years, there has been a renewed interest in the disease because of the increasing evidence of great clinical efficacy, on top of standard anticoagulant therapy, of adjunctive treatments such as pulmonary endarterectomy (PEA) [6] and, more recently, other approved treatments such as balloon pulmonary angioplasty (BPA) and advanced specific pharmacotherapy. This chapter summarises the diagnostic algorithm and the imaging examinations necessary in the evaluation of CTEPH.

2.2 Ventilation/Perfusion (V/Q) Lung Scan and Computed Tomography Pulmonary Angiography (CTPA)

A V/Q lung scan should be performed as the first exam when suspecting CTEPH because of its higher sensitivity compared with CTPA, especially in inexperienced centres [7]. The European Society of Cardiology guidelines on the diagnosis and management of acute pulmonary embolism support V/Q lung scan as the first-line test for diagnosing CTEPH following acute pulmonary embolism in the presence of dyspnoea or functional limitation [8]. A normal or low-probability V/Q lung scan can rules out CTEPH with a sensitivity of 90–100% and a specificity of 94–100% [1, 9]. In contrast, the presence of a high-probability V/Q lung scan makes CTEPH the most likely diagnosis, although other conditions may result in similar findings. A caveat is that unmatched perfusion defects may also be seen in other pulmonary vascular diseases such as pulmonary veno-occlusive disease (PVOD). Nevertheless, while for example in PVOD V/Q lung scan can show small peripheral unmatched and non-segmental perfusion defects, the typical findings of V/Q lung scan suggestive for CTEPH are at least one and often two or more major ventilation-perfusion mismatches (triangular segmental defects of perfusion) [10] (Fig. 2.1). Although some centres only perform a perfusion scan when searching for CTEPH, ventilation study is often useful in defining lung borders, aiding the detection of smaller peripheral perfusion defects. Moreover, ventilation scan provides additional information about alternative cardiopulmonary conditions, such as chronic obstructive lung disease and pneumonia. Therefore, the presence of even a single mismatched segmental perfusion defect in a patient with PH should raise concerns regarding a thromboembolic aetiology, but may result from non-embolic disorders, such as extrinsic vascular compression, pulmonary vasculitis, mediastinal fibrosis, pulmonary artery sarcoma or congenital pulmonary vascular abnormalities. It has to be kept in mind that the degree of perfusion scan abnormality can substantially understate the degree of actual obstruction deter-

mined angiographically or at surgery [11]. In a study of confirmed cases of CTEPH, V/Q lung scan was found to be superior to CTPA with a sensitivity of 97.4% versus 51% [7]. However, with the improvement of CTPA technology and interpretation skills, the difference between the two techniques has narrowed. Indeed, a more recent study has shown that both V/Q lung scan and CTPA are accurate methods for the detection of CTEPH with excellent diagnostic efficacy (100% sensitivity, 93.7% specificity and 96.5% accuracy for V/Q scan; 96.1% sensitivity, 95.2% specificity and 95.6% accuracy for CTPA) [9]. Planar V/Q lung scan identifies obstructions indirectly through V/Q mismatches whereas CTPA provides direct evidence of filling defects within vessels. In the setting of chronic obstructive pulmonary disease, the use of V/Q scan alone may be inappropriate for the correct diagnosis of CTEPH, due to possible confounding effects caused by air trapping and/or emphysema. In the daily practice of referral centres, both V/Q lung scan and CTPA are performed to achieve CTEPH diagnosis or, more generally, to identify a chronic thromboembolic disease: the first one because of the highest sensitivity, and the second for its higher specificity, especially for detecting vascular obstructions in lobar and segmental arteries

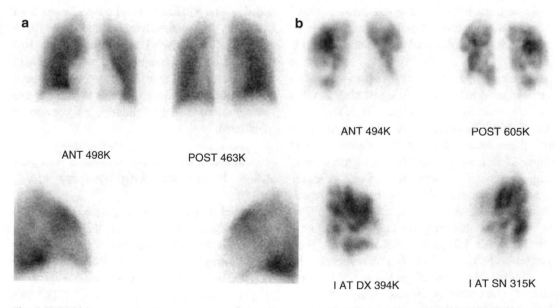

Fig. 2.1 (a) Normal perfusion lung scan; (b) multiple major defects of perfusion: high probability of CTEPH

[12]. In everyday clinical practice, CTPA is an easily available tool present in every medical centre and may demonstrate a variety of parenchymal, vascular or mediastinal abnormalities in patients with CTEPH [13]. Pulmonary abnormalities of CTEPH that can be seen on CTPA have been described extensively in the literature. The dilation of central pulmonary arteries with decreased diameter of peripheral vessels is a nonspecific sign, quite common in many PH patients, especially for those with a long history of the disease. Eccentric wall-adherent thrombi, which may be calcified, are more specific findings of CTEPH, very different from central filling defects within a distended lumen (the so-called polo mint sign), that are typical of acute pulmonary embolism. At the same time, the presence of a central thrombus on CTPA does not confirm the diagnosis of CTEPH, as it can be seen in other conditions (in situ thrombosis). Although not a specific feature, bronchial artery dilatation is frequently seen in CTEPH and has been shown to be associated with lower post-operative mortality and PVR after PEA [14]. Other abnormalities include mosaic parenchymal perfusion patterns (characterised by alternating regions of increased and decreased lung attenuation due to heterogeneous perfusion), parenchymal scars (due to prior pulmonary infarction), enlargement of the right ventricle, asymmetry in the size and distribution of lobar and segmental vessels, arterial webs or bands and mediastinal collateral vessels (Fig. 2.2). CTPA is currently widely used for the evaluation of operability because it can provide a vascular road map for surgical planning and it is the best modality for the delineation of the proximal cleavage plane for PEA [15]. Despite what guidelines recommend and the improvement in terms of technology, the infrequent use of V/Q lung scan in daily practice and the lack of expertise required to evaluate CTPA are still responsible for an underdiagnosis of CTEPH condition. In fact, it is still frequent that patients firstly referred to as idiopathic PAH may have their diagnosis changed to CTEPH after revaluation by an expert radiologist of previous CTPAs performed elsewhere. A correct interpretation of V/Q lung scan and CTPA holds not only diagnos-

tic but also therapeutic implications: a missed CTEPH diagnosis, for example, precludes lifelong anticoagulant therapy, which is mandatory in CTEPH. CTPA is adequate for the diagnosis of proximal CTEPH but a negative CTPA, even if high quality, does not exclude CTEPH as distal disease can be missed. Cone beam and area detector CT allow for more accurate visualisation of subsegmental vasculature and have been shown to be useful for procedural guidance for BPA. The benefits of the technology require validation in prospective trials before recommendation for routine clinical use.

2.3   3D Contrast-Enhanced Lung Perfusion MRI

3D contrast-enhanced lung perfusion MRI is a more recent and advanced imaging technique that can be deployed to search for perfusion defects in the pulmonary vascular bed. The advantage of MRI with respect to V/Q lung scan is that of improved spatial and temporal resolution, while with respect to CTPA it allows no radiation exposure for the patient. This is a major issue to be considered because diagnostic imaging investigations are usually performed within a few days from one another during hospital stay. A retrospective analysis has shown how perfusion MRI can reach similar sensitivity and specificity (97% and 92%, respectively) to that of CTPA [16]. Although being a reliable and safe diagnostic tool, its use is still restricted to specialised centres as faster and less expensive techniques are usually more widely available, as previously mentioned.

2.4   Pulmonary Angiography

High-quality pulmonary angiography, with or without digital subtraction, is still considered the gold standard for the diagnosis of CTEPH, especially when planning PEA or BPA, an alternative therapy for patients who are ineligible for PEA [17] or when V/Q lung scan and/or CTPA are inconclusive to confirm or to rule out CTEPH as

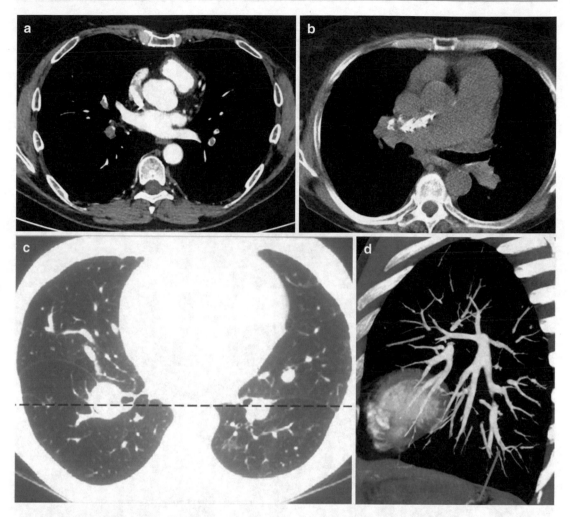

Fig. 2.2 (**a**) Polo mint candy sign in acute PE; (**b**) calcifications of pulmonary arteries; (**c**) variation in size of segmental vessels; (**d**) distal webs (green arrow)

the cause of PH. Due to the extreme complexity of the pulmonary vascular tree and to avoid huge amount of contrast medium, pulmonary angiography should be performed only in referral centres using a biplane angiographic system. In terms of angiographic technique, multiple selective injections are not required for the diagnosis of CTEPH whereas they could be essential for BPA. A single injection of non-ionic contrast into both proximal pulmonary arteries, with the volume and injection rate adjusted based on cardiac output, can provide sufficient anatomic detail. Biplane acquisition provides optimal anatomic detail, the lateral projection providing more detailed definition of lobar and segmental anat-

omy compared to the anteroposterior view alone (Fig. 2.3). Regarding diagnostic performance, Ley et al. showed in a prospective study that the sensitivity of conventional angiography was 66% at the main/lobar level and 76% at the segmental level, both of which were lower than that of CTPA [15]. Although being the gold standard for the diagnosis of CTEPH, pulmonary angiography is still an invasive and expensive tool. That being said, the overall complication rate is pretty low (0.9–4.8%) [18–20] but higher in case of severe PH and pulmonary artery dilation. Possible complications are related to the vascular access, to pulmonary vessel lesions (such as rupture or dissection) and ultimately to contrast agents.

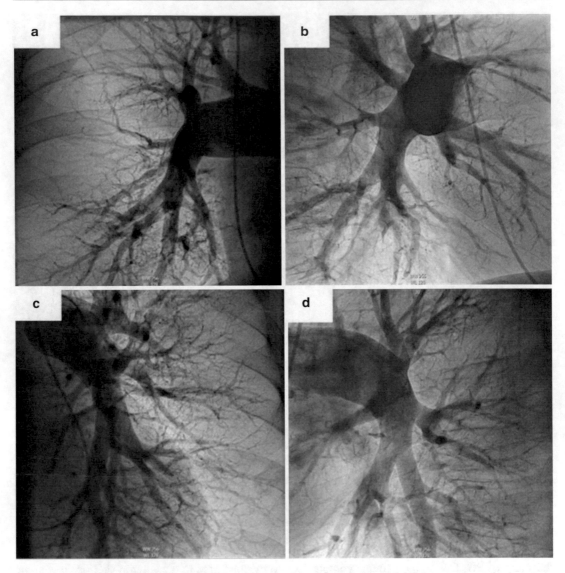

Fig. 2.3 Traditional pulmonary angiography showing multiple and bilateral segmental and subsegmental endoluminal filling defects. (**a**) Right-lung angiography in anteroposterior projection; (**b**) right-lung angiography in lateral-lateral view; (**c**) left-lung angiography in anteroposterior projection; (**d**) left-lung angiography in lateral-lateral view

Historically, five angiographic abnormalities have been described in CTEPH: (1) pouch defects; (2) pulmonary artery webs or bands; (3) intimal irregularities; (4) abrupt, often angular, narrowing of the major pulmonary arteries; and (5) complete obstruction of main, lobar or segmental vessels at their point of origin [21]. In such system, surgical findings were correlated with abnormal angiographic patterns obtained by a single injection of contrast medium into each main pulmonary artery with the catheter positioned in the main pulmonary arteries.

Distal lesions in peripheral pulmonary arteries were not visualised clearly by this method. Selective direct injection conventional angiography is widely available but requires expertise for use. In most patients with CTEPH, two or more of these angiographic findings are present, typically involving both lungs. The presence of different angiographic findings in the same patient, proximal and distal, some suitable for PEA, and others potentially treatable with BPA, and the degree of haemodynamic impairment that will be discussed later, can make multidisciplinary discussions on the best treatment for the patient very compelling. The vast majority of angiographic classifications of vascular lesions [21, 22] are based on specimens removed during PEA while there is little data on the angiographic features that can be used to identify the lesions best suitable for BPA. The need to update angiographic classifications for BPA's planning derives from the fact that organised thrombi are not removed during BPA and that the operator is able to evaluate lesions only by pulmonary angiographic images when performing BPA. Recently, Kawakami et al. proposed a novel angiographic classification of each vascular lesion in CTEPH based on selective angiograms and results of BPA [23]; a similar classification is used in coronary artery disease, where the definition of lesion type is based on the success rate of percutaneous coronary intervention [24]. Kawakami's classification describes five angiographic abnormalities: type A, ring-like stenosis lesion; type B, web lesion; type C, subtotal lesion; type D, total occlusion lesion; and type E, tortuous lesion [23]. Thromboembolic web-type lesions (type B of Kawakami's classification) were observed more frequently than the others, especially in lower lobes. Total occlusion (type D) and tortuous lesions (type E) were observed less frequently. Most thromboembolic lesions were located at the bifurcation of pulmonary artery branches, except for tortuous lesions [23]. Location and morphology of thromboembolic lesions also seem to affect the success and complication rate of BPA. Using Kawakami's classification, almost all BPA procedures were successful in ring-like stenosis and web lesions, whereas the success rates in total occlusion and tortuous lesions were only 52.2% and 63.6%, respectively. Moreover, the complication rate related to BPA (balloon injury, wire injury and perforation, and dissection of vessels) was higher for tortuous lesion (>40%) and subtotal lesions (15.5%) while <3% for ring-like stenosis and web lesions.

2.5 Right-Heart Catheterisation (RHC)

Given the complexity of pathophysiologic changes occurring in the pulmonary circulation in patients affected by CTEPH, after having investigated the presence, location and distribution of perfusion defects, it is mandatory to perform RHC to confirm the diagnosis of PH and to assess the degree of haemodynamic impairment. RHC is required to confirm the haemodynamic diagnosis of CTEPH and to distinguish it from chronic thromboembolic disease, which is characterised by similar symptoms and perfusion defects, but without PH at rest. Guidelines recommend a complete haemodynamic evaluation by RHC including cardiac output, because calculated PVR is important to assess the prognosis and risks associated with PEA [6]. Measurement of PAWP is necessary to exclude postcapillary PH resulting from comorbidities. Intravascular obstructions, such as the ones present in CTEPH, might confound the correct estimation of PAWP in some patients, and thus it is recommended to assess pulmonary arterial occlusion pressure in different vessels. When obtaining a good PAWP waveform is not possible, left ventricular end-diastolic pressure should be obtained by left ventricular catheterisation. Regarding the degree of haemodynamic impairment, it is necessary to bear in mind that there is an important difference in the behaviour of PVR between acute pulmonary embolism and CTEPH. In acute pulmonary embolism, there is a strong hyperbolic correlation between pulmonary vascular obstruction (PVO) and PVR, while most patients with CTEPH have higher PVR values than patients with acute PE for a given degree of PVO. This could probably be explained by the development of a microvasculopathy of vessels less than 500 μm in addition to the mechanical obstruction caused by proximal fibrotic obstruction in large elastic pulmonary arteries [25]. That being said, PVR and cardiac output are important parameters that have to be obtained before discussing the patient for surgery or for BPA. When performed at expert centres, RHC has low morbidity (1.1%) and mortality (0.055%) rates [26]. RHC is a technically demanding procedure that requires

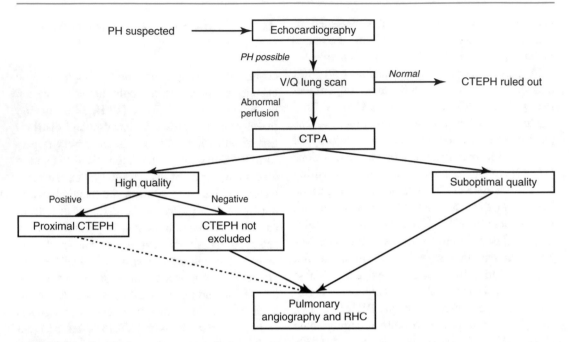

Fig. 2.4 CTEPH diagnostic algorithm used by expert centres in daily practice

meticulous attention to even the smallest detail to obtain clinically useful information. To obtain high-quality results with a low risk for the patient, the procedure should be limited to expert centres. Vasodilator testing does not appear to be useful or necessary in patients with CTEPH in determining operability, although preliminary data in a small cohort of patients suggest that preoperative vasodilator responsiveness (>10.4% reduction in mean pulmonary artery pressure) is associated with an improved long-term haemodynamic outcome in patients who subsequently undergo PEA [27].

Summarising recent data, the diagnostic algorithm for CTEPH that expert centres use in their practice is shown in Fig. 2.4.

CTEPH. Although V/Q lung scan is still considered the first-line screening modality, CTPA has become an important tool in the diagnostic workup, not only because it is able to show structural and vascular abnormalities, but also because it is able to rule out differential diagnoses. MRI provides both functional and physiological data in a single exam with great safety. High-quality pulmonary angiography is still necessary to confirm and define pulmonary vascular involvement and prior to making any treatment decision. It is usually performed in combination with RHC, which is mandatory to assess haemodynamics. In conclusion, the evolution of all diagnostic modalities is responsible for continuous improvement in the detection of CTEPH, which in turn may result in more favourable patient outcomes.

2.6   Conclusions

Imaging plays a central role in the diagnosis of CTEPH, a condition frequently under- or misdiagnosed in daily practice, but potentially curable with surgery or endovascular intervention. Noninvasive techniques are complementary and not competing modalities in the diagnosis of

References

1. Galiè N, et al. ESC/ERS guidelines for the diagnosis and treatment of pulmonary hypertension: the joint task force for the diagnosis and treatment of pulmonary hypertension of the European Society of Cardiology (ESC) and the European Respiratory Society (ERS) Endorsed by: Association for European Paediatric and Congenital Cardiology (AEPC), International

Society for Heart and Lung Transplantation (ISHLT). Eur Respir J. 2015;46(4):903–75. https://doi.org/10.1183/13993003.01032-2015.

2. Riedel M, Stanek V, Widimsky J, Prerovsky EI. Long-term follow-up of patients with pulmonary thromboembolism. Chest. 1982;81:151–8. https://doi.org/10.1378/chest.81.2.151.

3. Fedullo P, Kerr KM, Kim NH, Auger WR. Chronic thromboembolic pulmonary hypertension. Am J Respir Crit Care Med. 2011;183(12):1605–13. https://doi.org/10.1164/rccm.201011-1854CI.

4. Pepke-Zaba J, Hoeper MM, Humbert M. Chronic thromboembolic pulmonary hypertension: advances from bench to patient management. Eur Respir J. 2013;41(1):8–9. https://doi.org/10.1183/09031936.00181212.

5. Bonderman D, et al. Risk factors for chronic thromboembolic pulmonary hypertension. Eur Respir J. 2008;33(2):325–31. https://doi.org/10.1183/09031936.00087608.

6. Jenkins D, Madani M, Fadel E, D'Armini AM, Mayer E. Pulmonary endarterectomy in the management of chronic thromboembolic pulmonary hypertension. Eur Respir Rev. 2017;26:160111. https://doi.org/10.1183/16000617.0111-2016.

7. Tunariu N, et al. Ventilation-perfusion scintigraphy is more sensitive than multidetector CTPA in detecting chronic thromboembolic pulmonary disease as a treatable cause of pulmonary hypertension. J Nucl Med. 2007;48(5):680–4. https://doi.org/10.2967/jnumed.106.039438.

8. Konstantinides SV, et al. 2019 ESC Guidelines for the diagnosis and management of acute pulmonary embolism developed in collaboration with the European Respiratory Society (ERS). Eur Heart J. 2020;41(4):543–603. https://doi.org/10.1093/eurheartj/ehz405.

9. He J, et al. Diagnosis of chronic thromboembolic pulmonary hypertension: comparison of ventilation/perfusion scanning and multidetector computed tomography pulmonary angiography with pulmonary angiography. Nucl Med Commun. 2012;33(5):459–63. https://doi.org/10.1097/MNM.0b013e32835085d9.

10. Moser KM, Page GT, Ashburn WL, Fedullo PF. Perfusion lung scans provide a guide to which patients with apparent primary pulmonary hypertension merit angiography. West J Med. 1988;148(2):167–70.

11. Ryan KL, Fedullo PF, Davis GB, Vasquez TE, Moser KM. Perfusion scan findings understate the severity of angiographic and hemodynamic compromise in chronic thromboembolic pulmonary hypertension. Chest. 1988;93(6):1180–5. https://doi.org/10.1378/chest.93.6.1180.

12. Wang M, et al. Comparison of V/Q SPECT and CT angiography for the diagnosis of chronic thromboembolic pulmonary hypertension. Radiology. 2020;296(2):420–9. https://doi.org/10.1148/radiol.2020192181.

13. Shimizu H, et al. Dilatation of bronchial arteries correlates with extent of central disease in patients with chronic thromboembolic pulmonary hypertension. Circ J. 2008;72:1136. https://doi.org/10.1253/circj.72.1136.

14. Heinrich M, Uder M, Tscholl D, Grgic A, Kramann B, Schäfers H-J. CT scan findings in chronic thromboembolic pulmonary hypertension: predictors of hemodynamic improvement after pulmonary thromboendarterectomy. Chest. 2005;127(5):1606–13. https://doi.org/10.1378/chest.127.5.1606.

15. Ley S, et al. Diagnostic performance of state-of-the-art imaging techniques for morphological assessment of vascular abnormalities in patients with chronic thromboembolic pulmonary hypertension (CTEPH). Eur Radiol. 2012;22(3):607–16. https://doi.org/10.1007/s00330-011-2290-4.

16. Rajaram S, et al. 3D contrast-enhanced lung perfusion MRI is an effective screening tool for chronic thromboembolic pulmonary hypertension: results from the ASPIRE registry. Thorax. 2013;68(7):677–8. https://doi.org/10.1136/thoraxjnl-2012-203020.

17. Feinstein JA, Goldhaber SZ, Lock JE, Ferndandes SM, Landzberg MJ. Balloon pulmonary angioplasty for treatment of chronic thromboembolic pulmonary hypertension. Circulation. 2001;103(1):10–3. https://doi.org/10.1161/01.cir.103.1.10.

18. Zuckerman DA, Sterling KM, Oser RF. Safety of pulmonary angiography in the 1990s. J Vasc Interv Radiol. 1996;7(2):199–205. https://doi.org/10.1016/s1051-0443(96)70762-5.

19. Pitton MB, Kemmerich G, Herber S, Mayer E, Thelen M, Düber C. Hemodynamic effects of monomeric nonionic contrast media in pulmonary angiography in chronic thromboembolic pulmonary hypertension. Am J Roentgenol. 2006;187(1):128–34. https://doi.org/10.2214/AJR.04.0833.

20. Hofmann LV, et al. Safety and hemodynamic effects of pulmonary angiography in patients with pulmonary hypertension: 10-year single-center experience. Am J Roentgenol. 2004;183(3):779–85. https://doi.org/10.2214/ajr.183.3.1830779.

21. Auger WR, Fedullo PF, Moser KM, Buchbinder M, Peterson KL. Chronic major-vessel thromboembolic pulmonary artery obstruction: appearance at angiography. Radiology. 1992;182(2):393–8. https://doi.org/10.1148/radiology.182.2.1732955.

22. Thistlethwaite PA, et al. Operative classification of thromboembolic disease determines outcome after pulmonary endarterectomy. J Thorac Cardiovasc Surg. 2002;124:1203–11. https://doi.org/10.1067/mtc.2002.127313.

23. Takashi K, et al. Novel angiographic classification of each vascular lesion in chronic thromboembolic pulmonary hypertension based on selective angiogram and results of balloon pulmonary angioplasty. Circ Cardiovasc Interv. 2016;9:e003318. https://doi.org/10.1161/CIRCINTERVENTIONS.115.003318.

24. Ryan TJ, et al. Guidelines for percutaneous transluminal coronary angioplasty. A report of

the American College of Cardiology/American Heart Association Task Force on Assessment of Diagnostic and Therapeutic Cardiovascular Procedures (Subcommittee on Percutaneous Transluminal Coronary Angioplasty). Circulation. 1988;78(2):486–502. https://doi.org/10.1161/01. CIR.78.2.486.

25. Azarian R, et al. Lung perfusion scans and hemodynamics in acute and chronic pulmonary embolism. J Nucl Med. 1997;38:980.

26. Hoeper MM, et al. Complications of right heart catheterization procedures in patients with pulmonary hypertension in experienced centers. J Am Coll Cardiol. 2006;48:2546–52. https://doi.org/10.1016/j. jacc.2006.07.061.

27. Nika S-S, et al. Pulmonary vascular reactivity and prognosis in patients with chronic thromboembolic pulmonary hypertension. Circulation. 2009;119(2):298–305. https://doi.org/10.1161/ CIRCULATIONAHA.108.794610.

Pulmonary Thromboendarterectomy: The Only Cure for Chronic Thromboembolic Pulmonary Hypertension

3

D. P. Jenkins

3.1 Introduction

Pulmonary thromboendarterectomy: the only cure for CTEPH. In a book about balloon pulmonary angioplasty (BPA), this is a contentious statement with which to start a chapter. In addition, what is the definition of 'cure' that oncologists would suggest survival to 5 years, surgeons might suggest removal of visible obstructive material, and psychologists might indicate return to normal quality of life? In a disease defined by a haemodynamic threshold, the simplest definition of cure might be achievement of a mean pulmonary artery (PA) pressure < 25 mmHg. However, if we consider that PTE is the treatment with the longest duration of experience and evidence of efficacy, the treatment that can tackle disease from the pulmonary valve all the way to subsegmental pulmonary artery branches, and the current guideline-recommended treatment, then the statement begins to make more sense. In this chapter, I will discuss the evidence for pulmonary endarterectomy (PTE) as a cure for CTEPH, and where this surgical treatment differs from balloon pulmonary angioplasty (BPA). As with many major surgical procedures, this evidence is derived from case series and registries, as there has never been a randomized controlled trial of PTE surgery. However, of all the types of pulmonary hypertension, group 4 (CTEPH) is the cause that is most treatable today, and this is mainly because it is a macroscopic disease with obstructive pulmonary artery lesions that lend themselves to interventional rather than pharmaceutical therapies.

3.2 Historical Experience with PTE Surgery and Its Efficacy

Although sporadic attempts at pulmonary endarterectomy surgery occurred from the 1950s and later in the mid-1960s, the first case demonstrating reproducible long-term success and a thorough explanation of the disease management was published by the University of California at San Diego (UCSD) in 1973 [13]. By the 1990s the UCSD had refined the operation and begun performing a high volume of PTE surgery. This culminated in the first landmark surgical series published, 'Pulmonary endarterectomy: experience and lessons learned in 1500 cases' in 2003 [7]. This experience was further increased by a subsequent publication from the same institution extending this case series with another 500 patients from 2006 [11]. In terms of cumulative experience from a single institution, these case series remain the largest experience published. The series established that on average, PTE

D. P. Jenkins (✉)
Royal Papworth Hospital, Cambridge, UK
e-mail: david.jenkins1@nhs.net

© Springer Nature Switzerland AG 2022
F. Saia et al. (eds.), *Balloon pulmonary angioplasty in patients with CTEPH*,
https://doi.org/10.1007/978-3-030-95997-5_3

surgery could immediately reduce PVR to approximately 1/3 of preoperative values and mean PA pressure to just under ½ of the preoperative value, with a post-operative mean PA pressure of 26.0 mmHg for the most recent 500 cases. They comprehensively demonstrated both the utility and safety of PTE, but concentrated mainly on the perioperative short-term intrahospital outcomes.

In 2011, the surgical experience from the first international CTEPH registry was published [12]. This added 386 patients prospectively included in a predominantly European CTEPH registry, and operated at 17 surgical units. Again the reproducibility and success of the PTE treatment were confirmed. The importance of this publication was that the patients were prospectively included from diagnosis and that the surgical centres included smaller less experienced units. Thus, at the time of the fifth World Symposium in Pulmonary Hypertension in 2013, when the initial three reports describing successful BPA that emerged from Japan in 2012 were highlighted, there were already >3000 PTE cases reported in the world literature. Hence, whilst one treatment was emerging, the other was established and increasingly available and regarded as the only treatment proven to be successful at the time. It is important to understand that the patients reported in the surgical series described above were treated in an era before any licensed drug treatment for CTEPH was available.

In contrast to the relatively short-term outcomes described above, two further landmark publications were reported in Circulation in 2016 describing longer term outcomes from PTE surgery. These have confirmed the durability of the procedure and the sustained benefit on survival. The first described the follow-up of patients included in the first International CTEPH registry [3]. By 3-year follow-up, survival in the 404 operated patients was 89% compared with only 70% in the 275 patients who had not undergone PTE surgery. The second publication reported the 10-year follow-up of 880 patients from a complete national series from a single country (UK) [1]. At 10 years, survival was 72%, and survival improved by era as experience was gained. In the longer term, 40% of the deaths were due to unrelated causes, e.g. cancer. The detailed comprehensive programmed follow-up, with haemodynamic reassessment of patients post-PTE, also confirmed that only 49% met the strict haemodynamic definition of PA pressure < 25 mmHg at 3–6 months post-PTE. Therefore, one could argue that only half were 'cured', and that residual PH was relatively common. However, in this series, the residual PH appeared to be well tolerated, with a mean pulmonary artery pressure of ≥38 mmHg (PVR ≥425 dynes/sec/cm−5) required before it impacted on survival. Only 5 patients from the 880 had evidence of recurrent CTEPH.

There are multiple patient factors that determine the potential risk vs. benefit of PTE surgery. As this indicates, some PTE operations can be performed at low risk with a very high chance of a good outcome, whereas others may be both higher risk and give less predictable results. The latter procedures may be acceptable at a large experienced centre, but not at a less experienced one. There are few absolute contraindications to PTE surgery and as with mainly invasive large operations, those who are most sick have the most to gain.

A further factor to consider is what does cure mean to the patient. Doctors may worry about medium-term survival, haemodynamic changes and distances walked in an arbitrary 6 min, but for patients it is restoration of quality of life that is critical. Using the specific PH quality of life assessment tool CAMPHOR, it has been shown that there is dramatic improvement in quality of life post-PTE surgery. This improvement is proportional to the post-operative mean PA pressure [14]. Patients with a post-operative mean PA pressure < 30 mmHg had the most improvement and this was stable over 5-year follow-up.

This increasing experience of CTEPH treatment is mirrored by successive world PH symposia. At the fourth symposium in 2008, CTEPH did not merit a dedicated task force and the only accepted treatment was surgery. By the fifth symposium in 2013, CTEPH had gained a dedicated task force, and its own place in the PH classification, group 4, and BPA was mentioned as a possible new modality treatment [8]. By the sixth symposium in 2018, CTEPH retained its own task force and the focus was on multimodality treatment with three possibilities [9].

3.3 Nature and Distribution of the Disease

Preoperative imaging can provide a good indication of the type and level of disease found at the time of surgery, but it is far from exact and remains only an estimate. The actual distribution of clearable disease, and the ease of the dissection plane, is only confirmed at the time of surgery when both the patient and surgeon are already committed to the treatment. This is the underlying reason why operability assessment is difficult in this disease. It is the surgeon alone who gets the direct feedback from correlating the preoperative imaging to the material cleared at surgery and the immediate haemodynamic benefit.

The pathology of CTEPH has been described in detail [4] but there are many factors that we still do not understand. Why does CTEPH develop in the first place, when the majority of patients get complete resolution post-acute pulmonary embolism? Why do some patients remain stable for many years, whereas others with an apparent similar burden of disease deteriorate rapidly? Why do some pulmonary circulations retain compliance protecting the right ventricle, but others do not?

The morphology of the disease that the surgeon encounters within the pulmonary arteries is highly variable too, and is dependent on the degree of clot lysis, amount of organization and position that the original acute clots were trapped (see Fig. 3.1). The variation exists between patients and even within the same patient. At the most proximal level there can be total occlusion of a main pulmonary artery or partial obliteration with bulky laminated thrombus. At the other end of the surgical extreme, there may be normal endothelium all the way down to subsegmental branching with distal occlusive webs in vessels only 1–2 mm in diameter. Distal segmental and subsegmental disease can be cleared by an experienced surgeon with good results [2]. The technical procedure is a true endarterectomy where a plane is created within the PA wall and the obstructive material removed from the circulation. This necessitates cardiopulmonary bypass, cooling to 20 °C and periods of deep hypothermic circulatory arrest to allow the surgeon clear view deep into the PA branches [10]. Thus surgery offers the greatest range of lesions that can be cleared and material that can be removed at multiple sites within the PA tree. There is undoubtedly a degree of overlap of which disease can be reached and treated by BPA and PTE, but the threshold for one versus the other is not easily demarcated on imaging and is operator dependent. The haemodynamic impact is determined by the percentage of the pulmonary circulation opened, and the effect on PVR, rather than the bulk of the disease removed.

The classification of surgical disease is an intraoperative one that cannot be determined from preoperative imaging. The original (Jamieson) classification described four types of disease, with a suggestion that type 4 was not CTEPH at all [15]. A more recent revision describes levels 1–4 from the main PA to subsegmental level rather than type of disease.

3.4 What Do the Guidelines Recommend?

The latest joint ESC/ERS guidelines on the treatment of pulmonary hypertension were published in 2016 [5]. These gave a 1C recommendation for PTE surgery as the treatment for CTEPH. The class of recommendation at 1 was the highest, but the level of evidence was only C as there has not been a RCT or meta-analysis. At the sixth world symposium in PH, the treatment algorithm for CTEPH was simplified and divided patients with CTEPH into 'operable' and 'non-operable' [9]. For operable patients the clear recommendation was PTE surgery, and this was designated the treatment of choice. Non-operable patients were recommended targeted medical therapy, with or

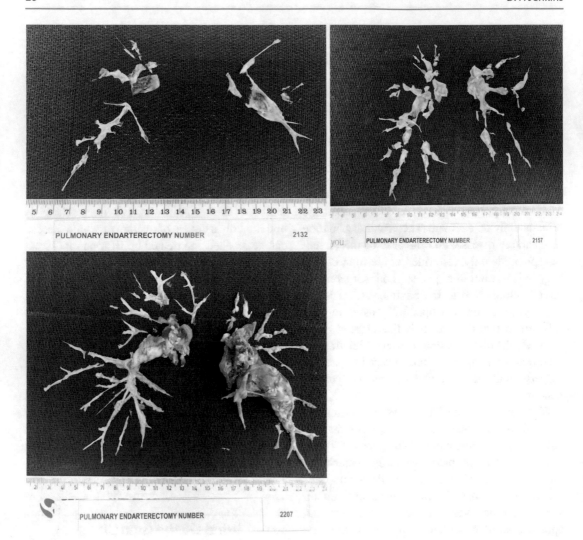

Fig. 3.1 Examples of pulmonary endarterectomy, excised specimens arranged anatomically, demonstrating the range of disease from more distal to proximal

without BPA, and this reflected the evidence from the CHEST-1 RCT study [6].

3.5 Why PTE? Fundamental Differences Between PTE Surgery and BPA

In summary, I would suggest that the benefits of PTE surgery include the following:

• Ability to actually remove the physical disease from the PA.

• Ability to treat all types and most levels of disease.
• A 'one-stop' treatment with immediate haemodynamic improvement.

Overall the most evidence to date for improvements that translate into longer term survival and quality of life for patients.

However, unlike BPA, PTE requires a general anaesthetic, sternotomy incision, intensive care and a prolonged recovery period.

As with all treatment decisions, it is a trade-off between risk and benefit for the patient and ultimately the patient needs to make the decision.

The parallels are similar to the treatment of coronary artery disease with coronary artery bypass surgery or percutaneous stenting. The most invasive procedure is likely to give the most comprehensive improvement that is longer lasting, but at the expense of more upfront risk. If any treatment of CTEPH deserves the label of 'cure' then PTE surgery remains the front runner for the majority of patients. However, it is increasingly recognized that some patients may require multimodality treatment with all three therapies to get the best long-term result.

References

1. Cannon JE, Su L, Kiely DG, Page K, Toshner M, Swietlik E, et al. Dynamic risk stratification of patient long-term outcome after pulmonary endarterectomy: results from the United Kingdom National Cohort. Circulation. 2016;133(18):1761–71.
2. D'Armini AM, Morsolini M, Mttiucci G, et al. Pulmonary endarterectomy for distal chronic thromboembolic pulmonary hypertension. J Thorac Cardiovasc Surg. 2014;148:1005–11.
3. Delcroix M, Lang I, Pepke-Zaba J, Jansa P, D'Armini AM, Snijder R, et al. Long-term outcome of patients with chronic thromboembolic pulmonary hypertension: results from an international prospective registry. Circulation. 2016;133(9):859–71.
4. Dorfmuller P, Gunther S, Ghigna M-R, et al. Microvascular disease in chronic thromboembolic pulmonary hypertension: a role for pulmonary veins and systemic vasculature. Eur Respir J. 2014;44:1275–88.
5. Galie N, Humbert M, Vachiery JL, Gibbs S, Lang I, Torbicki A, et al. 2015 ESC/ERS guidelines for the diagnosis and treatment of pulmonary hypertension: the joint task force for the diagnosis and treatment of pulmonary hypertension of the European Society of Cardiology (ESC) and the European Respiratory Society (ERS): endorsed by: Association for European Paediatric and Congenital Cardiology (AEPC), International Society for Heart and Lung Transplantation (ISHLT). Eur Heart J. 2016;37(1):67–119.
6. Ghofrani HA, D'Armini AM, Grimminger F, Hoeper MM, Jansa P, Kim NH, et al. Riociguat for the treatment of chronic thromboembolic pulmonary hypertension. N Engl J Med. 2013;369(4):319–29.
7. Jamieson SW, Kapelanski DP, Sakakibara N, et al. Pulmonary endarterectomy: experience and lessons learned in 1,500 cases. Ann Thorac Surg. 2003;76:1457–62.
8. Kim N, Delcroix M, Jenkins DP, Channick R, Dartevelle P, Jansa P, et al. Chronic thromboembolic pulmonary hypertension. J Am Coll Cardiol. 2013;62:92–9.
9. Kim NH, Delcroix M, Jais X, Madani MM, Matsubara H, Mayer E, et al. Chronic thromboembolic pulmonary hypertension. Eur Respir J. 2019;53(1):1801915.
10. Madani M, Mayer E, Fadel E, Jenkins DP. Pulmonary endarterectomy. Patient selection, technical challenges, and outcomes. Ann Am Thorac Soc. 2016;3:240–7.
11. Madani MM, Auger WR, Pretorius V, et al. Pulmonary endarterectomy: recent changes in a single institution's experience of more than 2,700 patients. Ann Thorac Surg. 2012;94:97–103.
12. Mayer E, Jenkins D, Lindner J, et al. Surgical management and outcome of patients with chronic thromboembolic pulmonary hypertension: results from an international prospective registry. J Thorac Cardiovasc Surg. 2011;141:702–10.
13. Moser KM, Braunwald NS. Successful surgical intervention in severe chronic thromboembolic pulmonary hypertension. Chest. 1973;64:29–35.
14. Newnham M, Bunclark K, Abraham N, Ali S, Amaral-Almeida L, Cannon JE, et al. CAMPHOR score: patient-reported outcomes are improved by pulmonary endarterectomy in chronic thromboembolic pulmonary hypertension (CTEPH). Eur Respir J. 2020; https://doi.org/10.1183/13993003.02096-2019.
15. Thistlethwaite PA, Mo M, Madani MM, Deutsch R, Blanchard D, Kapelanski DP, et al. Operative classification of thromboembolic disease determines outcome after pulmonary endarterectomy. J Thorac Cardiovasc Surg. 2002;124(6):1203–11.

Medical Treatment of Chronic Thromboembolic Pulmonary Hypertension

4

Nick H. Kim

4.1 Introduction

The treatment of chronic thromboembolic pulmonary hypertension (CTEPH) has evolved to a multimodal approach including the use of PH-targeted medical therapy. The rationale and accumulating data in support of medical therapy will be reviewed. Unanswered questions in CTEPH in need of investigation and careful consideration include the role of these medical therapies.

4.2 Anticoagulation

Following the diagnosis of chronic thromboembolic pulmonary hypertension (CTEPH), medical management begins with effective lifelong anticoagulation [1]. Traditionally, this has been with oral vitamin K antagonist therapy, with routine monitoring to ensure safe and effective dosing. With the availability of direct oral anticoagulants (DOACs) which offer convenient advantages over vitamin K antagonist therapy (VKA), this added convenience is offset by limited experience in the setting of CTEPH [2, 3]. Up to 20% of CTEPH patients can have concomitant antiphos-

pholipid antibody syndrome [4]—representing a substantial portion of CTEPH patients who may not be ideal candidates for DOACs [5]. A retrospective analysis from the UK also highlighted concerns with the use of DOACs in CTEPH [6]. In patients followed after pulmonary endarterectomy, 206 patients maintained on DOACs were noted to have a higher incidence of recurrent thrombotic complications compared to the group of 794 patients on vitamin K antagonist. The rates of thrombotic complications for the DOAC group were 4.62%/patient-year versus just 0.76%/patient-year for the VKA group. A single-center retrospective review from a high-volume pulmonary endarterectomy (PEA) program in the USA found that patients on chronic DOAC therapy prior to PEA were two times more likely than VKA counterparts to have acute or subacute clot discovered at the time of PEA [7]. Despite limitations from these retrospective analyses, there remains some preliminary concern that CTEPH patients may respond differently to DOACs compared with traditional VKA. In summary, although evidence is lacking to guide detailed anticoagulation management in CTEPH under varying treatment conditions, in general the anticoagulation strategy should mirror that of venous thromboembolism treatment with the additional caveat and caution regarding the subgroup of CTEPH patients with antiphospholipid antibody syndrome.

N. H. Kim (✉)
Division of Pulmonary, Critical Care, and Sleep Medicine, University of California,
San Diego, CA, USA
e-mail: h33kim@ucsd.edu

© Springer Nature Switzerland AG 2022
F. Saia et al. (eds.), *Balloon pulmonary angioplasty in patients with CTEPH*,
https://doi.org/10.1007/978-3-030-95997-5_4

4.3 PH-Targeted Therapy

The rationale in support of PH-targeted medical therapy in CTEPH includes histopathological observations and an unmet clinical need for a substantial subgroup of CTEPH patients (Table 4.1). Plexogenic lesions, previously felt to be unique to idiopathic pulmonary arterial hypertension (PAH), have been described in lung biopsies obtained from patients with CTEPH [8, 9]. The presence of these and other small-vessel changes in CTEPH patients undergoing PEA did not appear to preclude beneficial results of surgery [8]. Plausible links to small-vessel changes in CTEPH have come from abnormalities in vasoactive compounds previously described in PAH. For example, elevated circulating levels of the nitric oxide synthase inhibitor asymmetric dimethylarginine and elevated endothelin-1 levels have each been reported in patients with CTEPH [10, 11]. However, the component of small-vessel disease may be more complicated than previously appreciated based on the subsequent report elaborating systemic to pulmonary collateral circulation, and even venous and capillary involvement in select cases with severe treatment-refractory CTEPH leading to death or lung transplantation [12]. Experimental preoperative measures to predict patients with a significant degree of small-vessel disease have been reported, but not routinely available for operability or treatment assessment [13, 14].

The unmet clinical need in CTEPH was highlighted by two important reports. In the international CTEPH registry conducted across the EU

Table 4.1 Rationale for investigating PH-targeted medical therapy for the treatment of CTEPH

Similar microvascular arteriopathy as seen in pulmonary arterial hypertension (PAH)
Abnormalities in circulating endothelin-1 and inhibitors of nitric oxide synthase
Uncontrolled reports of benefit from all three pathways of PAH therapeutics
Nearly 40% of CTEPH cases deemed inoperable
Nearly half of the patients followed up after PEA have residual pulmonary hypertension
Facilitation of high-risk interventional treatment (PEA or BPA) with combination/bridging approach

and one center in Canada, up to 40% of CTEPH patients, even among these experienced surgical centers, were deemed not candidates for pulmonary endarterectomy [15, 16]. Furthermore, the national CTEPH registry from the UK revealed that up to half of the patients following PEA can have residual PH on follow-up right-heart catheterization [17]. Lastly, with the advances in PAH-targeted medical treatments, there were numerous uncontrolled reports of compassionate or experimental use of these therapies with observed benefit in CTEPH. The evidence with PH-targeted medical therapy, however, is drawn from the following important randomized controlled trials (RCT).

4.4 AIR Study (Inhaled Iloprost)

The first prospective RCT for inoperable CTEPH was the AIR study investigating the effects of the inhaled prostacyclin analog iloprost [18]. Two groups were studied, idiopathic PAH group versus other forms of PH combining scleroderma-associated PAH and anorexigen-associated PAH, along with 57 patients with inoperable CTEPH. The groups were randomized between inhaled iloprost treatment and placebo for a duration of 12 weeks. The primary endpoint was a composite of 6-min walk distance (6MWD) improvement by $\geq 10\%$ from baseline, together with improvement in New York Heart Association functional class, without clinical worsening or death. The combined primary endpoint was observed in 20.8% receiving iloprost compared to 5.5% in the placebo group for the idiopathic PAH subgroup. For the other PH group including CTEPH, iloprost treatment was associated with 12.5% reaching the primary endpoint versus 4.3% for the placebo group. The key limitations of this study from the standpoint of CTEPH outcomes are lack of an operability adjudication process and lack of subgroup analysis of the CTEPH cohort in response to iloprost. Based on the results of this trial, inhaled iloprost was approved for the treatment of PAH but not for inoperable CTEPH (https://www.accessdata.fda.gov/drugsatfda_docs/nda/2004/21-779_Ventavis_approv.pdf).

4.5 BENEFIT Study (Oral Bosentan)

The first dedicated RCT for inoperable CTEPH was the BENEFIT study with the dual-endothelin receptor antagonist bosentan [19]. Adult CTEPH patients deemed to have technically inoperable disease or patients with persistent PH >6 months after PEA were eligible for this multicenter, prospective, double-blind study of bosentan therapy. All cases deemed inoperable were reviewed in a post hoc manner by a panel of experts including 2 PEA surgeons and 2 CTEPH specialists. Of the 157 enrolled patients, 28% had prior PEA with persistent PH. Patients were randomized to either bosentan or placebo for a duration of 16 weeks. Independent co-primary endpoints were changes from baseline to week 16 in PVR and 6MWD. At the end of 16 weeks, the bosentan-treated group saw a treatment effect of −24.1% in PVR (95% CI, −31.5 to −16.0; P <0.0001). However, this did not translate into improvements in exercise capacity as measured by 6MWD (treatment effect +2.2 m) (95% CI, −22.5 to 26.8; P = 0.5449). A reason for this discrepancy between the efficacy endpoints was postulated as relating to 16 weeks potentially not being an adequate duration to see an exercise capacity improvement. An example of this was observed in a small pilot study with sildenafil in CTEPH; 6MWD failed to show improvement at the primary endpoint analysis time point of 12 weeks, but showed improvement when followed out to 12 months [20]. In addition to the duration of study endpoint being potentially important for CTEPH, the importance of operability adjudication was emphasized in this study and served as a reminder for future medical treatment studies in CTEPH.

4.6 CHEST-1 Study (Oral Riociguat)

The first positive RCT of a PH-targeted medical therapy in CTEPH was CHEST-1 [21]. Riociguat is an orally available soluble guanylate cyclase stimulator which increases the production of cyclic GMP resulting in, among other effects, vasodilation of the pulmonary circulation. CHEST-1 was a prospective, double-blind, randomized study of technically inoperable CTEPH and patients with persistent/recurrent CTEPH following PEA. Operability assessment was incorporated prospectively prior to randomization by either a central committee of CTEPH experts or approved local adjudication centers based on experience [22]. Patients were randomized to either riociguat (n = 173) or placebo (n = 88) for 16-week duration. The primary endpoint was changed in 6MWD from baseline at week 16. The results were positive in favor of riociguat titrated up to a maximum dose of 2.5 mg taken orally three times daily. The treatment effect was +46 m gain (95% CI, 25 to 67; P < 0.001) at 16 weeks with sustained separation from the placebo group notable by week 8. The riociguat group also improved key secondary endpoints including PVR reduction, NT-proBNP reduction, and functional class improvement by week 16. Although both the technically inoperable and post-PEA groups improved with riociguat, the trend was greater with the technically inoperable group. Patients completing CHEST-1 were eligible to enter the long-term open-label study CHEST-2. Of the 237 patients in CHEST-2, the improvements in 6MWD were maintained out to 2 years. No new treatment-related adverse events were found. Observed survival at 2 years was 93% (95% CI, 89 to 96) with a clinical worsening-free survival of 82% (95% CI, 77 to 87) while on riociguat therapy. The main limitations of CHEST-1 were the exclusion of other PH-targeted therapies and the exclusion of balloon pulmonary angioplasty (BPA).

4.7 MERIT Study (Oral Macitentan)

MERIT-1 was a prospective phase 2 RCT investigating the effects of macitentan 10 mg daily in patients with technically inoperable CTEPH [23]. A prospective adjudication of operability was utilized. Background non-parenteral PH targeted therapy was allowed provided the therapy was stable for at least

1 month prior to study inclusion (61% enrolled on background therapy). Post-PEA patients or those undergoing BPA procedures were excluded. The primary endpoint was PVR reduction at week 16. Change in 6MWD from baseline was the first of hierarchical secondary endpoints and was not measured until week 24. A total of 80 patients were randomized to either placebo or macitentan 10 mg daily. At week 16, both groups observed a drop from baseline PVR; however, the macitentan group saw a treatment effect in PVR reduction by 16% (0.84; 95% CI 0.70-0.99, p=0.041). At week 24, the macitentan treatment effect on 6MWD was +34.0 m (95% CI 2.9-65.2, p-0.033) in favor of macitentan treatment. No new safety signal was reported that has not been previously observed with macitentan. This was the first RCT in CTEPH to allow for background therapy. However, 1 month may not have been an adequate minimum stable duration of background therapy based on the placebo group also improving in the primary analysis. Macitenan is currently being investigated in a phase 3 study for inoperable CTEPH (https://clinicaltrials.gov; NCT04271475).

4.8   CTREPH Study (Subcutaneous Treprostinil)

Subcutaneous treprostinil infusion was investigated in a phase 3 trial for patients with CTEPH who were not treatable with PEA for a variety of reasons [24]. A total of 105 patients were enrolled between 2009 and 2016, randomized to receive either low dose (target dose 3 ng/kg/min) or higher dose (target dose 30 ng/kg/min) subcutaneous treprostinil infusion prior to assessment at week 24. The primary endpoint at week 24 was change from baseline 6MWD. The treatment effect in favor of higher dose infusion was +40.69 m (95% CI 15.86–65.53, $p = 0.0016$). Secondary endpoints of functional class improvement, PVR reduction, and NT-proBNP reduction were also in favor of the higher dose group. Site

pain was reported in 74% of the higher dose group (1 discontinuation) and 81% of the low-dose group (3 discontinuations). Based on these results, EMA approved the use of subcutaneous treprostinil for the treatment of inoperable CTEPH (https://www.ema.europa.eu/en/medicines/human/EPAR/trepulmix).

4.9   Medical Therapy in Combination with Other Treatment Modalities

PH-targeted medical therapy is unlikely to target the proximal mechanical component of CTEPH treated with either PEA or BPA [25]. Accordingly, combining PH-targeted medical therapy and either interventions has been the subject of interest and investigations. The concept of bridging high-risk, severe CTEPH cases with PH-targeted medical therapy prior to PEA was initiated but abandoned due to slow enrollment and challenges with the COVID-19 pandemic (https://clinicaltrials.gov; NCT03273257). In the absence of data, the current consensus opinion is to avoid delaying PEA (for cases deemed operable) with a trial of unproven PH-targeted therapy [26]. The combination of PH-targeted medical therapy and BPA, however, has garnered more appeal with some emerging data in favor of such a combination strategy. Most patients undergoing BPA treatment also meet the indication for PH-targeted medical therapy [1, 27]. The soon-to-be-published RACE study will include valuable data on patients receiving both BPA and riociguat therapies in its crossover design [28].

The evaluation and treatment of CTEPH are now multidisciplinary and multimodality processes that require expertise coming together from PEA surgery, BPA interventionists, PH specialists, and radiology [26, 27]. There are numerous gaps in our understanding of PH-targeted medical therapy in the treatment of CTEPH (Table 4.2). Current and future investigations, as well as real-world registries, should offer some clarity and direction for future inquiries.

Table 4.2 Key unanswered questions for the role of PH-targeted medical therapy in CTEPH

Monotherapy vs. combination medical therapy
Safety and efficacy of bridging severe operable CTEPH cases prior to PEA
Effect of PH medical therapies on specimen integrity at the time of PEA
Target threshold for optimizing the first BPA with PH-targeted medical therapy
Continuation or cessation of PH-targeted medical therapy with BPA treatments
Variable response within CTEPH subgroups to treatments including PH therapy

4.10 Conclusion

Medical treatment of CTEPH begins with effective lifelong anticoagulation. For operable CTEPH, PEA is recommended without delay. For those patients who are deemed inoperable, or cases with persistent/recurrent PH after PEA, PH-targeted medical therapies are available and may be used in conjunction with BPA.

References

1. Galiè N, Humbert M, Vachiery JL, et al. 2015 ESC/ERS guidelines for the diagnosis and treatment of pulmonary hypertension: the joint task force for the diagnosis and treatment of pulmonary hypertension of the European Society of Cardiology (ESC) and the European Respiratory Society (ERS): endorsed by: Association for European Paediatric and Congenital Cardiology (AEPC), International Society for Heart and Lung Transplantation (ISHLT). Eur Respir J. 2015;46:903–75.
2. Gavilanes F, Alves JL Jr, Fernandes CJC, et al. The use of new anticoagulants in CTEPH. Eur Respir J. 2017;50:2409. https://doi.org/10.1183/1393003.congress-2017.
3. Sena S, Bulent M, Derya K, et al. Real-life data of direct anticoagulant use, bleeding risk and venous thromboembolism recurrence in chronic thromboembolic pulmonary hypertension patients: an observational retrospective study. Pulm Circ. 2020;10:2045894019873545.
4. Wolf M, Boyer-Neumann C, Parent F, et al. Thrombotic risk factors in pulmonary hypertension. Eur Respir J. 2000;15:395–9.
5. Ghembaza A, Saadoun D. Management of antiphospholipid syndrome. Biomedicine. 2020;8:508.
6. Bunclark K, Newnham M, Chiu YD, et al. A multicenter study of anticoagulation in operable chronic thromboembolic pulmonary hypertension. J Thromb Haemost. 2020;18:114–22.
7. Jeong I, Fernandes T, Alotaibi M, Kim NH. Direct oral anticoagulant use and thrombus detection in patients with chronic thromboembolic pulmonary hypertension referred for pulmonary endarterectomy. Eur Respir J. 2019;54:OA5161. https://doi.org/10.1183/13993003.congress-2019.
8. Moser KM, Bloor CM. Pulmonary vascular lesions occurring in patients with chronic major vessel thromboembolic pulmonary hypertension. Chest. 1993;103:685–92.
9. Yi ES, Kim H, Ahn H, et al. Distribution of obstructive intimal lesions and their cellular phenotypes in chronic pulmonary hypertension. A morphometric and immunohistochemical study. Am J Respir Crit Care Med. 2000;162:1577–86.
10. Skoro-Sajer N, Mittermayer F, Panzenboeck A, et al. Asymmetric dimethylarginine is increased in chronic thromboembolic pulmonary hypertension. Am J Respir Crit Care Med. 2007;176:1154–60.
11. Reesink HJ, Meijer RC, Lutter R, et al. Hemodynamic and clinical correlates of endothelin-1 in chronic thromboembolic pulmonary hypertension. Circ J. 2006;70:1058–63.
12. Dorfmuller P, Gunther S, Ghigna MR, et al. Microvascular disease in chronic thromboembolic pulmonary hypertension: a role for pulmonary veins and systemic vasculature. Eur Respir J. 2014;44:1275–88.
13. Kim NHS, Fesler P, Channick RN, et al. Preoperative partitioning of pulmonary vascular resistance correlates iwth early outcome after thromboendarterectomy for chronic thromboembolic pulmonary hypertension. Circulation. 2004;109:18–22.
14. Toshner M, Suntharalingam J, Fesler P, et al. Occlusion pressure analysis role in partitioning of pulmonary vascular resistance in CTEPH. Eur Respir J. 2012;40:612–7.
15. Pepke-Zaba J, Delcroix M, Lang I, et al. Chronic thromboembolic pulmonary hypertension (CTEPH): results from an international prospective registry. Circulation. 2011;124:1973–81.
16. Delcroix M, Lang I, Pepke-Zaba J, et al. Long-term outcome of patients with chronic thromboembolic pulmonary hypertension (CTEPH): results from an international prospective registry. Circulation. 2016;133:859–71.
17. Cannon JE, Su L, Kiely DG, et al. Dynamic risk stratification of patient long-term outcome after pulmonary endarterectomy: results from the UK national cohort. Circulation. 2016;133:1761–71.
18. Olschewski H, Simonneau G, Galie N, et al. Inhaled iloprost for severe pulmonary hypertension. N Engl J Med. 2002;347:322–9.
19. Jais X, D'Armini AM, Jansa P, et al. Bosentan for treatment of inoperable chronic thromboembolic pulmonary hypertension: BENEFiT (Bosentan effects in iNopErable forms of chronIc thromboembolic pulmonary hypertension), a randomized, placebo-controlled trial. J Am Coll Cardiol. 2008;52:2127–34.

20. Suntharalingam J, Treacy CM, Doughty NJ, et al. Long-term use of sildenafil in inoperable chronic thromboembolic pulmonary hypertension. Chest. 2008;134:229–36.

21. Ghofrani HA, D'Armini AM, Grimminger F, et al. Riociguat for the treatment of chronic thromboembolic pulmonary hypertension. N Engl J Med. 2013;369:319–29.

22. Jenkins DP, Biederman A, D'Armini AM, et al. Operability assessment in CTEPH: lessons from the CHEST-1 study. J Thorac Cardiovasc Surg. 2016;152:669–74.

23. Ghofrani HA, Simonneau G, D'Armini AM, et al. Macitentan for the treatment of inoperable chronic thromboembolic pulmonary hypertension (MERIT-1): results from the multicentre, phase 2, randomised, double-blind, placebo-controlled study. Lancet Respir Med. 2017;5:785–94.

24. Sadushi-Kolici R, Jansa P, Kopec G, et al. Subcutaneous treprostinil for the treatment of severe non-operable chronic thromboembolic pulmonary hypertension (CTREPH): a double-blind, phase 3, randomised controlled trial. Lancet Respir Med. 2019;7:239–48.

25. Simonneau G, Torbicki A, Dorfmuller P, Kim N. The pathophysiology of chronic thromboembolic pulmonary hypertension. Eru Respir Rev. 2017;26:160112.

26. Delcroix M, Torbicki A, Gopalan D, et al. ERS statement on chronic thromboembolic pulmonary hypertension. Eur Respir J. 2020;2020:2002828.

27. Kim NH, Delcroix M, Jais X, et al. Chronic thromboembolic pulmonary hypertension. Eur Respir J. 2019;53:1801915.

28. Jaïs X, Brenot P, Bouvaist H, et al. Late breaking abstract – balloon pulmonary angioplasty versus riociguat for the treatment of inoperable chronic thromboembolic pulmonary hypertension: results from the randomised controlled RACE study. Eur Respir J. 2019;54:RCT1885. https://doi.org/10.1183/13993003.congress-2019.

Balloon Pulmonary Angioplasty in Chronic Thromboembolic Pulmonary Hypertension: Modern Technique

Hiromi Matsubara and Aiko Ogawa

5.1 Patient Selection and Preparation for BPA

All symptomatic patients with chronic thromboembolic pulmonary hypertension (CTEPH) diagnosed as inoperable by a multidisciplinary CTEPH team could be candidates for balloon pulmonary angioplasty (BPA) [1]. Those include not only patients with surgically inaccessible lesions but also patients with inoperable conditions due to comorbidities. Patients with residual or recurrent pulmonary hypertension after pulmonary endarterectomy could also be candidates for BPA [2]. Hemodynamic severity and advanced age are not generally considered contraindications [3]. In cases with severe renal dysfunction, the risk/benefit ratio should be considered. The sole contraindication for BPA is patients with a serious iodine allergy, which cannot be controlled by immunosuppressants [4]. Symptomatic patients with chronic thromboembolic pulmonary disease without pulmonary hypertension may also be candidates for BPA, though there are only reports of a few case series [5, 6].

Global pulmonary angiography (Fig. 5.1a) and lung perfusion scans (Fig. 5.1b) should be performed before BPA to evaluate the distribution of the thromboembolic lesions. Alternatively, dual-energy computed tomography can be used instead of perfusion scans. Preselection of the initial target lobe (right or left) should be decided based on the distribution of the perfusion defects and lesion types (for further detail of lesion types, please see Chap. 7). All lesions should be targets because the current aim of BPA is total revascularization. However, the preselection of all target lesions is both unnecessary and unlikely as it is difficult to recognize all of the lesions without selective pulmonary angiography. Generally, all segmental pulmonary arteries have some lesions (Fig. 5.1c–f), though the severity of blood flow impairment in each segmental pulmonary artery (PA) varies.

Anticoagulants are continued during the BPA procedure to maintain a prothrombin time-international ratio between 2.0 and 3.0. Alternatively, it can be substituted by heparin. Before starting BPA procedures, 500–2000 units of heparin is administered to reach an activated clotting time of approximately 200 seconds. Pulmonary hypertension-targeted drugs can be continued if the drugs were prescribed prior to BPA [7]. However, given the time and cost, initiation of these drugs shortly before BPA is dispensable [8], though they might be effective in reducing the risk of complications after

H. Matsubara (✉)
Department of Cardiology, National Hospital Organization Okayama Medical Center, Okayama, Japan

A. Ogawa
Department of Clinical Science, National Hospital Organization Okayama Medical Center, Okayama, Japan

© Springer Nature Switzerland AG 2022
F. Saia et al. (eds.), *Balloon pulmonary angioplasty in patients with CTEPH*,
https://doi.org/10.1007/978-3-030-95997-5_5

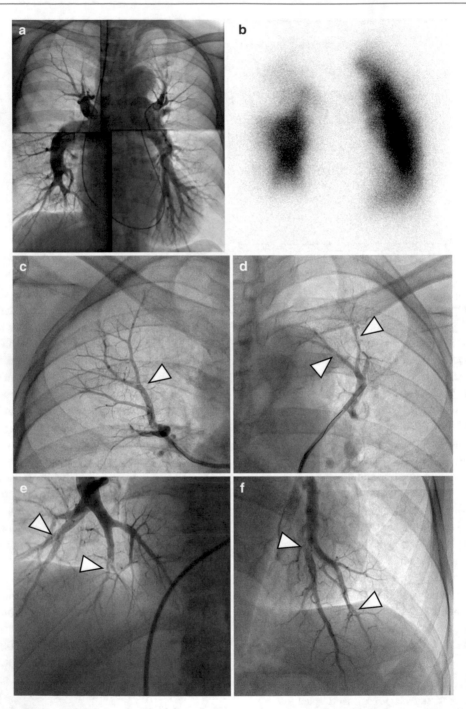

Fig. 5.1 Representative case of a 71-year-old woman with inoperable chronic thromboembolic pulmonary hypertension (CTEPH) before balloon pulmonary angioplasty. (**a**) Global pulmonary angiogram (PAG) of the patient. Segmental pulmonary arteries appear to be intact. Lesions in the subsegmental arteries are hard to recognize. (**b**) Perfusion scans of the patient. Perfusion defects are observed predominantly in the right lung. (**c**) Selective PAG of the apical segmental artery of the right upper lobe (A1). Web lesion (arrowhead) is seen at the bifurcation of the subsegmental arteries. (**d**) Selective PAG of the apical segmental artery of the left upper lobe (A1). Web lesions (arrowhead) are noted at the bifurcations of the distal-subsegmental arteries. (**e**) Selective PAG of the lateral (left side) and posterior (right side) segmental arteries of the right lower lobe (A9 and 10). Web lesions (arrowhead) are seen at the bifurcations of the subsegmental arteries in both segmental arteries. (**f**) Selective PAG of the posterior segmental artery of the left lower lobe (A10). Web lesions (arrowhead) are observed at the bifurcations of the subsegmental and distal-subsegmental arteries

BPA. According to our experience, 5 L/min oxygen inhalation via mask could immediately decrease the mean PA pressure of CTEPH patients by around 10%, without changing the cardiac output. This reduction in mean PA pressure achieved by oxygen inhalation is comparable to that of targeted drugs, while the additional time and cost are minimal. Administering supplemental oxygen immediately before BPA sufficiently reduces the risk of complications.

Most BPA procedures can be performed via a femoral approach. Existence of a permanent caval filter does not impede BPA if the inferior vena cava is patent. In specific cases, such as caval occlusion or total occlusion of the proximal right PA in which a strong backup force is crucial, approach from the right jugular vein is inevitable. Generally, a 6 Fr or 7 Fr system is better than an 8 Fr system for delivery and manipulation of the guiding catheter. For smooth manipulation or changing of the guiding catheter, a long sheath, which can reach the bilateral main PA, is recommended. A standard 9 Fr outer sheath makes it easy to manipulate the tip of the long sheath. In cases with total occlusion of the proximal PA, an 8 Fr system is required to generate the backup force necessary to penetrate the occluded site (for understanding the BPA for proximal lesions, please see Chap. 9).

5.2 BPA Procedures

5.2.1 Selection and Angiogram of Segmental PAs

It is crucial to select the guiding catheter based on the shape of branching in each segmental PA. Generally, the Judkins right catheter is useful for all segmental PAs. However, after entering each segmental PA, it cannot be positioned coaxial to the lesions, which complicates the passage of the guidewire to the lesions, except for arteries in the upper lobe. The shapes of frequently used guiding catheters suitable for each segmental PA are shown in Table 5.1. We commonly use a multipurpose-type guiding catheter for the right PA and an Amplatz left-type guiding catheter for

Table 5.1 Compatibility of guiding catheters with each segmental artery

Segment	JL-4		JR-4		AL-1		MP	
	R	L	R	L	R	L	R	L
A1	×	×	◎	◎	○	○	○	△
A2*	×	×	◎	◎	○	○	○	○
A3	×	◎	◎	△	○	○	○	△
A4	×	◎	○	△	○	○	◎	△
A5	×	◎	○	△	◎	○	○	△
A6	×	×	○	○	△	○	◎	◎
A7**	△	×	○	○	◎	○	△	◎
A8	×	×	○	△	○	◎	◎	○
A9	×	×	○	○	○	◎	◎	○
A10	×	×	○	○	△	◎	◎	○

◎ best, ○ good, △ possible, × bad.
AL Amplatz left, *JL* Judkins left, *JR* Judkins right, *MP* multipurpose.
* Although the posterior part of the left upper lobe is part of the apico-posterior segment, the pulmonary artery usually has a separate branch perfusing it.
** The artery going to this part is frequently found as a large branch of A6 and occasionally as a branch of A8 or A10, despite the absence of a medial segment of the left lower lobe.

the left PA. After advancing the guiding catheter into the segmental PA, selective pulmonary angiography is essential for a precise evaluation of the lesion characteristics [9]. The tip of the guiding catheter should be positioned as close as possible to the lesion to obtain precise information of the lesion distal vessels. Further, 3–4 ml of contrast medium diluted with saline (contrast: saline = 2:1 to 3:1) is enough to obtain a clear image. Due to the multitude of small branches overlapping the lesion, obtaining at least two images from different directions is recommended as reference images. Utilization of a biplane angiography system helps reduce the amount of contrast medium. Having patients hold their breath upon deep inspiration straightens the segmental PA and facilitates recognition of the lesion characteristics, especially those of the lower lobe.

5.2.2 Passing the Lesions with Guidewire

After obtaining reference images of the target vessel, a 0.014-inch guidewire is used to pass the lesion. Commonly used wires for coronary or peripheral artery interventions can be used. However, considering the high incidence of vascular injury during BPA procedures caused by the tip of the guidewire [10], hard-tip guidewires with more than a 3 g tip load should be avoided. Deep insertion of the guidewire into the subsegmental PA is usually difficult because of the limited length of the subsegmental PA. The highly flexible radiopaque distal end of a guidewire longer than 30 mm is not suitable for BPA because of the loss of support for passing balloon catheters. Furthermore, slippery guidewires can advance too far into the distal small branches and may injure them. Thus, hydro-coated guidewire tips are also generally not recommended for BPA. To overcome these issues, we developed a custom guidewire dedicated for BPA (B-pahm 0.6, Japan Lifeline Co., Ltd., Tokyo, Japan). The tip load of this guidewire is only 0.6 g and the highly flexible distal end of the wire is only

20 mm. It does not enter into the small branches because the 10 mm distal end has no hydro-coating, and it rarely causes vascular injury.

It is difficult to pass severely stenotic lesions using a soft-tip guidewire without hydro-coating. Thus, we frequently use a balloon catheter for assistance in passing such a lesion. In this technique, a 2.0 mm diameter balloon catheter is used to increase the backup force, similar to using a microcatheter. When the wire bends at the proximal end of the lesion to become a large knuckle shape (Fig. 5.2a, b), the balloon catheter is advanced until it contacts the lesion (Fig. 5.2c). The wire is straightened by pulling back and can then enter the channel within the lesion (Fig. 5.2d, e). When the wire is stuck within the lesion (Fig. 5.2f, g), proceeding the balloon catheter until its tip enters into the lesion (Fig. 5.2h) and then pushing the wire can make the knuckle shape and enable the wire to enter into the large channel (Fig. 5.2i, j). Although the backup force obtained by the balloon catheter is smaller

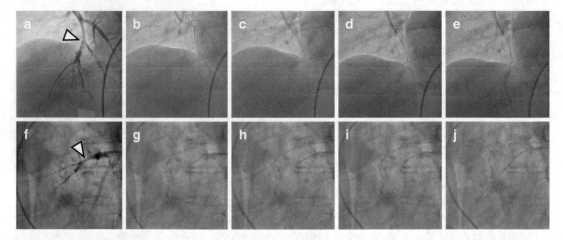

Fig. 5.2 Representative images of passing the lesion with the balloon catheter-assisted guidewire in the same case shown in Fig. 5.1. The second procedure of right A10 (a–e) and left A3 (F-J) is shown. (a) Selective pulmonary angiogram (PAG) of the posterior segmental artery of the right lower lobe (A10) one month after the initial balloon pulmonary angioplasty (BPA) with a 2 mm balloon. Lesion (arrowhead) and lesion distal vessels were enlarged compared to those before BPA (Fig. 5.1e). (b) The guidewire (B-pahm 0.6, Japan Lifeline Co., Ltd., Tokyo, Japan) could not pass the lesion and became a large knuckle shape. (c) A balloon catheter (Pulcone™ 3.0–4.0 × 20 mm, NIPRO, Osaka, Japan) was advanced until it contacted the lesion. (d) After pulling back, the guidewire straightened

and was able to enter the channel within the lesion. (e) Guidewire and balloon catheter could pass the lesion. (f) Selective PAG of the anterior segment of left upper lobe (A3) 1 month after the initial BPA with a 2 mm balloon. The web lesion (arrowhead) was observed just proximal to the bifurcation of the subsegmental arteries. (g) The guidewire used in the right A10 stuck within the lesion and could not pass the lesion. (h) A balloon catheter (Pulcone™ 2.0–3.0 × 20 mm, NIPRO, Osaka, Japan) was advanced until its tip entered into the lesion. (i) Pushing the guidewire with the support of the balloon catheter made the guidewire knuckle shaped, and it was able to enter the largest channel in the lesion. (j) Guidewire passed the lesion while keeping the knuckle shape than that of a microcatheter, it is usually enough to pass severely stenotic lesions. By eliminating the use of a microcatheter, we can diminish cost and procedural time. Having patients holding their breath upon deep inspiration aids in passing the lesions, especially those in the lower lobe.

5.2.3 Balloon Dilation in Stenotic Lesions: Sizing

During our initial experience, the diameter of the balloon was chosen based on PA angiogram reference images, and we tried to fully dilate the lesions during the initial dilation, as in coronary interventions [11]. As a result, many BPA procedures resulted in bloody sputum and lung injury. The lesions in CTEPH are composed mainly of fibrous tissues [12, 13] and are much harder than coronary plaques. The relatively rough meshwork structure of the web lesion is prone to disruption by balloon dilation. However, the lesions' solid and tight component could not be compressed by balloon dilation. The vessel wall of a normal PA is thinner than that of a systemic artery and thus, stretching the original PA vessel walls enables fundamental lumen enlargement after BPA [14]. Full dilation, aiming for complete elimination of the stenosis, would cause overdilation with stretch and injury to vessel walls, and result in oozing hemorrhage from the dilated sites, especially in severely stenotic lesions with a greater amount of fibrous tissues [13]. After understanding this pathophysiology of lumen enlargement in BPA, we limited the balloon size according to the intravascular ultrasound (IVUS). The balloon diameter was decided as 50–80% of the vessel diameter measured by IVUS, based on the amount of fibrous tissues in the lesion and PA pressure. Although this strategy could diminish the occurrence of vascular injury caused by balloon dilation [15], it increases the risk of vascular injury caused by the wire tip as it is a complex procedure requiring a frequent change of devices. In addition, IVUS observation could not be obtained in about 30% of the lesions before BPA [14], meaning that this strategy is not a perfect solution for eliminating the occurrence of vascular injury.

After starting BPA with a smaller balloon size, spontaneous enlargement, instead of restenosis, of the residual stenosis at the lesion was commonly observed [16] (Fig. 5.3a–d), thus making stent implantation dispensable. It seemed that increasing blood flow through the lesion was more important than increasing the internal pressure at the lesion, because internal pressure at the lesion immediately after BPA was almost the same as before BPA in most cases. Based on our preliminary observation, for all lesions, small balloons, such as those with a 2.0 mm diameter, were sufficient to induce spontaneous enlargement of the stenotic lesions by restoring the minimal blood flow through the lesion. Therefore, we use 2.0 mm diameter balloons for the initial treatment of all lesions, irrespective of the vessel diameter. In case of unsatisfactory restoration of blood flow and low PA pressure (<40 mmHg), up to a 3.0 mm diameter balloon can be used. Then, 1–3 months after the initial dilation, patients undergo repeat dilation of all lesions with appropriate balloon diameters (3.0–6.0 mm) to finalize the intervention (Fig. 5.4). Importantly, in the second dilation, balloon size should be selected based on the vessel diameter just proximal to the lesions to optimize the result (Fig. 5.3e, f).

5.2.4 Balloon Dilation in Stenotic Lesions: Other Tips

Generally, balloon catheters used for coronary or peripheral intervention can be used for BPA. Balloons around 20 mm in length are sufficient to cover the lesion length. If the balloon catheter cannot pass the lesion, reconfirmation of the guidewire position by checking images from a different direction is recommended. Usually, passing the balloon catheter through the lesion is not difficult, even when passing the guidewire was difficult. The guidewire may enter an extremely small branch overlapping the target segmental PA. In the initial treatment of segmental PAs, only the critical lesion should be dilated, even if there appears to be other distal vessel

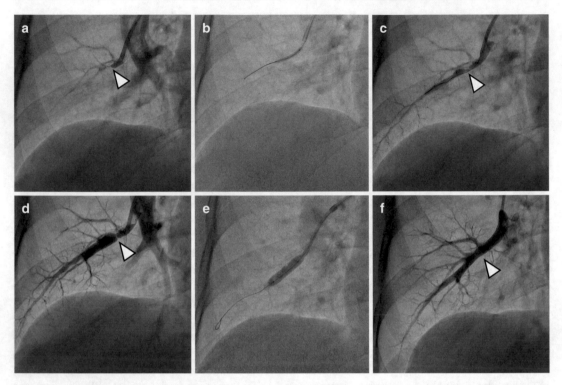

Fig. 5.3 Representative images of spontaneous enlargement of the treated lesion after balloon pulmonary angioplasty. (**a**) Selective pulmonary angiogram (PAG) of the anterior segment of the right lower lobe (A8) revealed a subtotal occlusion lesion (arrowhead). (**b**) The initial dilation of the lesion with a small balloon (Ikazuchi 2.0 × 20 mm, Kaneka Medix Corporation, Osaka, Japan). (**c**) Selective PAG of the right A8 after the initial dilation. Stenosis (arrowhead) remains after revascularization of the distal artery. (**d**) Selective PAG of the right A8 1 month after the initial dilation. The lesion (arrowhead) and lesion distal vessels were spontaneously enlarged without additional dilation. (**e**) The second dilatation of the lesion with a large balloon (Aviator 5.5 × 20 mm, Cordis/Cardinal Health Japan, Tokyo, Japan) to optimize the dilation. (**f**) One year after the second dilation of the lesion. Stenosis is completely abolished at the previously occluded site (arrowhead)

lesions; vessels, distal to the critical lesion, have been protected from high PA pressure and are prone to vascular injury caused by dilation.

In cases with steep tapering of the original vessel diameter with web-type lesions, it is difficult to decide the balloon size. Dilation of the lesion, using the proximal reference for the balloon diameter, frequently causes vascular injury at the distal end of the lesion. In contrast, balloon diameters, using the distal reference, would be insufficient to dilate the lesion. To solve this problem, we developed a tapered balloon (Pulcone™ 2.0–3.0 × 20 mm or 3.0–4.0 × 20 mm, NIPRO, Osaka, Japan). The diameter of the balloon is tapered from 3.0 mm to 2.0 mm or 4.0 mm to 3.0 mm within a 20 mm length (Fig. 5.5). It is useful not only in avoiding vascular injury but

also in reducing the number of balloon catheters used during the procedure because vessel diameters between 2.0 mm and 4.0 mm can be covered with only two catheters.

5.2.5 Treatment of Total and Subtotal Occlusion Lesions

Subtotal occlusion lesions are considered as the most severely stenotic web lesions [9, 14]. Treatment for subtotal occlusion lesions is basically the same as those for web lesions. The guiding catheter tip should be strictly positioned coaxially to the lesion; a daughter catheter might be helpful to correct the direction of the guiding

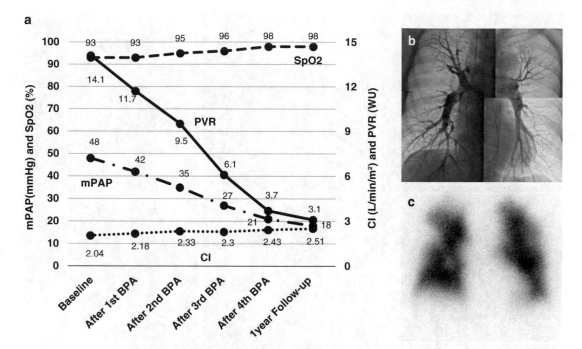

Fig. 5.4 Representative case with inoperable CTEPH (shown in Fig. 5.1) treated by BPA. (**a**) Clinical course of the case with mean pulmonary artery pressure (mPAP), cardiac index (CI), pulmonary vascular resistance (PVR), and oxygen saturation in ambient air (SpO₂). All segmental arteries were treated, except for right A4, for which we could not find the occluded orifice. All parameters were normalized after four BPA procedures. In the initial BPA, 12 lesions in the right lung were treated for 46-min radiation time using 75 ml of contrast medium and a 2.0 mm diameter balloon. In the second BPA, performed 5 days after the initial BPA, 13 lesions in the left lung were treated for 32-min radiation time using 80 ml of contrast medium and a 2.0 mm diameter balloon. In the third BPA, performed 1 month after the second BPA, 15 lesions in the right lung were treated for 37-min radiation time using 80 ml of contrast medium and two balloon catheters (3.0–

4.0 and 5.5 mm diameter). In the fourth BPA, performed the day after the third BPA, 19 lesions in the left lung were treated for 45-min radiation time using 105 ml of contrast medium and two balloon catheters (2.0–3.0 and 3.0–4.0 mm diameters). Even using only a 2.0 mm diameter balloon, both the hemodynamics and SpO₂ sufficiently improved by treating multiple lesions. Note that an expert operator can complete BPA procedures quickly with minimal contrast medium. (**b**) Global pulmonary angiogram 1 year after the final BPA. The pulmonary arteriogram is almost normal compared to before BPA (Fig. 5.1a). (**c**) Perfusion scans 1 year after the final BPA. Perfusion defects almost completely disappeared, except for the right A4. Note that the entire effect of BPA is excellent (Fig. 5.4a) although one segmental artery was left untreated

catheter tip. Usually, passing the lesion with a soft-tip guidewire supported by a balloon catheter is not difficult. Occasionally, a hard-tip wire with hydro-coating is necessary. In such cases, however, simultaneous usage of microcatheter is not recommended because the backup force is too strong, increasing the danger of vascular injury.

Total occlusion lesions existing at the subsegmental PAs are also treatable with standard techniques using soft-tip guidewires. To obtain a

backup force sufficient to penetrate the lesions, support with a balloon catheter or microcatheter is required. When using hard-tip wires with hydro-coating, special attention should be paid not to insert the guidewire deeply to avoid vascular injury at the distal vessel, because of the short length of the subsegmental PAs and the multitude of adjacent small branches. Increasing the backup force with simultaneous usage of a microcatheter and hard-tip guidewire to penetrate total occlusion lesions in the subsegmental PAs would be

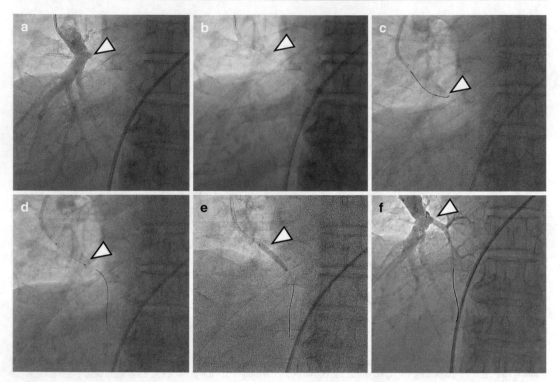

Fig. 5.5 Representative images of BPA for total occlusion lesion at the orifice of the medial segmental artery of the right lower lobe (A7). (**a**) Angiogram indicated the unnatural bend of the right basal PA without branching and stump (arrowhead) of probable A7. (**b**) Although the tip of the Judkins right-type guiding catheter was correctly directed to the stump (arrowhead), engagement was impossible. (**c**) A guidewire with a 2 g tip load and hydrophilic coating (Chevalier 14 Floppy BPA, NIPRO, Osaka, Japan) supported by a balloon catheter (Pulcone™ 2.0–3.0 x 20 mm, NIPRO, Osaka, Japan) could proceed to the stump (arrowhead). (**d**) The hard-tip guidewire could pass the occluded lesion (arrowhead). (**e**) Dilation of the lesion (arrowhead) with a balloon catheter. A tapered balloon (3.0 mm to 2.0 mm) within 20 mm length was used. (**f**) Selective pulmonary angiography after balloon dilation of the lesion (arrowhead) showed revascularization of A7

harmful as in subtotal occlusion lesions. Microcatheters are useful only when changing to a softer guidewire after passing the lesion.

Total occlusion lesions located at the orifice of segmental or subsegmental arteries might be difficult to recognize for beginners. They can be recognized by finding the avascular area, which should be perfused by the target segmental PAs. The silhouette of the target segmental or subsegmental PA might facilitate location of the target vessels. The existence of an unnatural bend of the lobar or segmental PA (Fig. 5.5a) signifies the entry of the totally occluded segmental or subsegmental PA. Once operators recognize the lesions, passing the guidewire in total occlusion lesions at the orifice of subseg-

mental PAs is not difficult. However, in cases with total occlusion lesions at the orifice of segmental PAs, BPA procedures are intractable because engaging the guiding catheter to the segmental PAs is extremely challenging. Although the direction of the guiding catheter tip can be set by specific shape selection, such as a curve for the internal mammalian artery or short Amplatz, sufficient backup force is hard to obtain (Fig. 5.5b). To penetrate lesions with fibrous tissues totally covering the entry of the target vessels, simultaneous usage of a hard-tip guidewire with hydro-coating and a microcatheter is necessary (Fig. 5.5c–f).

Total occlusion lesions existing at the proximal segmental PAs or proximal PAs are vastly different from those existing at more distal PAs. Usually, these lesions have a typical "pouch" appearance and are hard to penetrate with ordinary techniques (for further detail of the treatment for proximal lesions, please see Chap. 9).

5.2.6 Number of Target Lesions in a Procedure

To obtain a greater improvement in hemodynamics, it is essential to restore PA blood flow to as normal as possible. It is known that the more segments are treated, the greater the improvement in patient hemodynamics [11]. Therefore, the total revascularization of CTEPH patients is the final treatment goal of BPA. However, it is impossible to accomplish it with only a single procedure. Thus, we divided the BPA treatment into several procedures, with specific end points for each procedure. We limited the dosage of contrast medium to within 200 ml and the radiation time to within 60 minutes for each procedure. In more than 800 BPA procedures during the past 5 years in our hospital, the average dosage of the contrast medium and radiation time per procedure were 80 ml and 35 minutes, respectively [8].

The treatment of lesions causing large perfusion defects and obstructive lesions (i.e., total occlusion and subtotal occlusion lesions), rather than stenotic lesions, effectively increases the effect of the procedure. Conversely, these efforts might increase the risk of potentially life-threatening complications. The number and type of target lesions within a procedure should be decided based on the patients' hemodynamic severity and operators' skill. Previously, we treated only stenotic lesions in the initial procedure because they are generally easy to treat, and the number of treated lesions was around 4 [11]. Currently, we treat all of the lesions within the unilateral lung (10–15 lesions) including occlusive lesions, irrespective of the patients' hemodynamic severity. Usually, our current BPA treatment can be completed with 4–5 procedures even though we are adopting staged dilation for all lesions (Fig. 5.4).

5.2.7 Recognition and Treatment of Complications

Even with carefully performed procedures, complete prevention of complications is impossible because of the nature of the treatment and disease. Thus, we must prepare for the inevitable occurrence of complications. During the procedure, the key complication to avoid is vascular injury and caution for the resultant hemorrhage is warranted after occurrence [10]. The details of the diagnosis and management of vascular injury are described in Chap. 11. Briefly, it can be recognized by the following four signs: new onset of cough with or without bloody sputum, elevation of heart rate more than 20 bpm, oxygen desaturation more than 5%, and extravasation of contrast medium during the angiogram. Any vascular injury left untreated may cause massive bleeding or lung injury after BPA and thus should be treated during BPA procedures. The basic treatment for vascular injury is to stop bleeding by proximally occluding the injured vessels. Since the aim of BPA is to restore the blood flow of all target PAs, temporal occlusion of the target PA with balloons or gelatin embolization, rather than a permanent occlusion, such as a coil embolization, is preferred [17].

5.3 Treatment Goal and Follow-Up

The final treatment goal of BPA in our center is to achieve a resting mPAP less than 25 mmHg and an oxygen saturation under ambient air greater than 95% [8]. To reach this treatment goal, all segmental arteries are systematically treated. However, some segmental PAs appear to be untreatable with BPA. This number of segmental PAs will decrease as operators' skill in finding absent segmental PAs improves. The important point is to treat as many lesions as possible. After completing BPA for all treatable lesions, we usually perform patient follow-ups 6 months after the final BPA procedure, and then every year for 5 years. Currently, approximately 70% of the patients reach the treatment goal by the 6-month follow-up in our center. Once the patients reach the treatment goal, recurrence of hemodynamic impairment is extremely rare up to 5 years, if sufficient anticoagulation is continued. Thus, annual follow-up with right-heart catheterization might not be mandatory in such cases after 5 years. Careful follow-up is a requisite because deterioration of symptoms or hemodynamics was observed in about half of those who had not reached the treatment goal at the 6-month follow-up.

5.4 Conclusion

For the past 18 years, we have continuously refined the BPA procedure to establish the treatment strategy and techniques described above. As a result, BPA has become a standard treatment for inoperable CTEPH patients in our center. As BPA prevails worldwide as an alternative treatment for CTEPH patients who are deemed inoperable, we hope that our modern BPA techniques help improve its efficacy and safety.

References

1. Kim NH, Delcroix M, Jais X, Madani MM, Matsubara H, Mayer E, et al. Chronic thromboembolic pulmonary hypertension. Eur Respir J. 2019;53:1.
2. Shimura N, Kataoka M, Inami T, Yanagisawa R, Ishiguro H, Kawakami T, et al. Additional percutaneous transluminal pulmonary angioplasty for residual or recurrent pulmonary hypertension after pulmonary endarterectomy. Int J Cardiol. 2015;183:138–42.
3. Yanagisawa R, Kataoka M, Inami T, Shimura N, Ishiguro H, Fukuda K, et al. Safety and efficacy of percutaneous transluminal pulmonary angioplasty in elderly patients. Int J Cardiol. 2014;175(2):285–9.
4. Fukuda K, Date H, Doi S, Fukumoto Y, Fukushima N, Hatano M, et al. Guidelines for the treatment of pulmonary hypertension (JCS 2017/JPCPHS 2017). Circ J. 2019;83(4):842–945.
5. Wiedenroth CB, Olsson KM, Guth S, Breithecker A, Haas M, Kamp JC, et al. Balloon pulmonary angioplasty for inoperable patients with chronic thromboembolic disease. Pulm Circ. 2018;8(1):2045893217753122.
6. Inami T, Kataoka M, Kikuchi H, Goda A, Satoh T. Balloon pulmonary angioplasty for symptomatic chronic thromboembolic disease without pulmonary hypertension at rest. Int J Cardiol. 2019;289:116–8.
7. Wiedenroth CB, Ghofrani HA, Adameit MSD, Breithecker A, Haas M, Kriechbaum S, et al. Sequential treatment with riociguat and balloon pulmonary angioplasty for patients with inoperable chronic thromboembolic pulmonary hypertension. Pulm Circ. 2018;8(3):2045894018783996.
8. Ogawa A, Matsubara H. After the dawn-balloon pulmonary angioplasty for patients with chronic thromboembolic pulmonary hypertension. Circ J. 2018;82(5):1222–30.
9. Kawakami T, Ogawa A, Miyaji K, Mizoguchi H, Shimokawahara H, Naito T, et al. Novel angiographic classification of each vascular lesion in chronic thromboembolic pulmonary hypertension based on selective angiogram and results of balloon pulmonary angioplasty. Circ Cardiovasc Interv. 2016;9:10.
10. Ejiri K, Ogawa A, Fujii S, Ito H, Matsubara H. Vascular injury is a major cause of lung injury after balloon pulmonary angioplasty in patients with chronic thromboembolic pulmonary hypertension. Circ Cardiovasc Interv. 2018;11(12):e005884.
11. Mizoguchi H, Ogawa A, Munemasa M, Mikouchi H, Ito H, Matsubara H. Refined balloon pulmonary angioplasty for inoperable patients with chronic thromboembolic pulmonary hypertension. Circ Cardiovasc Interv. 2012;5(6):748–55.
12. Chausheva S, Naito A, Ogawa A, Seidl V, Winter MP, Sharma S, et al. Chronic thromboembolic pulmonary hypertension in Austria and Japan. J Thorac Cardiovasc Surg. 2019;158(2):604–14.
13. Kitani M, Ogawa A, Sarashina T, Yamadori I, Matsubara H. Histological changes of pulmonary arteries treated by balloon pulmonary angioplasty in a patient with chronic thromboembolic pulmonary hypertension. Circ Cardiovasc Interv. 2014;7(6):857–9.
14. Shimokawahara H, Ogawa A, Mizoguchi H, Yagi H, Ikemiyagi H, Matsubara H. Vessel stretching is a cause of lumen enlargement immediately after balloon pulmonary angioplasty: intravascular ultrasound analysis in patients with chronic thromboembolic pulmonary hypertension. Circ Cardiovasc Interv. 2018;11(4):e006010.
15. Kurzyna M, Darocha S, Pietura R, Pietrasik A, Norwa J, Manczak R, et al. Changing the strategy of balloon pulmonary angioplasty resulted in a reduced complication rate in patients with chronic thromboembolic pulmonary hypertension. A single-centre European experience. Kardiol Pol. 2017;75(7):645–54.
16. Nagayoshi S, Ogawa A, Matsubara H. Spontaneous enlargement of pulmonary artery after successful balloon pulmonary angioplasty in a patient with chronic thromboembolic pulmonary hypertension. EuroIntervention. 2016;12(11):e1435.
17. Inami T, Kataoka M, Shimura N, Ishiguro H, Yanagisawa R, Kawakami T, et al. Incidence, avoidance, and management of pulmonary artery injuries in percutaneous transluminal pulmonary angioplasty. Int J Cardiol. 2015;201:35–7.

Balloon Pulmonary Angioplasty for Chronic Thromboembolic Pulmonary Hypertension: Clinical Outcomes

6

Irene M. Lang

Abbreviations

6-MWD	6-Minute walking distance
BPA	Balloon pulmonary angioplasty
CI	Cardiac index
CI	Confidence interval
CO	Cardiac output
CTED	Chronic thromboembolic disease
CTEPH	Chronic thromboembolic pulmonary hypertension
CTO	Chronic total occlusion
Dlco	Diffusion capacity for carbon monoxide
ECMO	Extracorporeal membrane oxygenation
eGFR	Estimated glomerular filtration rate
mPAP	Mean pulmonary artery pressure
NT-proBNP	N-terminal pro-brain natriuretic peptide
OR	Odds ratio
PAG	Pulmonary angiography
PEA	Pulmonary endarterectomy
PH	Pulmonary hypertension
PVR	Pulmonary vascular resistance
QoL	Quality of life
RAP	Right atrial pressure
RCT	Randomized controlled trial
WHO	World Health Organization

I. M. Lang (✉)
Department of Internal Medicine II, Division of Cardiology, Vienna General Hospital, Medical University of Vienna, Vienna, Austria
e-mail: irene.lang@meduniwien.ac.at

6.1 Introduction

Chronic thromboembolic pulmonary hypertension (CTEPH) is characterized by major vessel pulmonary vascular lesions that are the sequelae of thrombi which obstruct flow in large vessels of the pulmonary circulation. In 40% of cases these lesions are accompanied by microvascular disease which is a predictor of postoperative outcome after pulmonary endarterectomy (PEA) [1]. In 15% of patients microvascular disease is visible as poor subpleural perfusion on pulmonary angiograms (PAG), and is associated with decreased response to balloon pulmonary angioplasty (BPA) [2]. In the porcine model, microvascular lesions may be transient and disappear if pulmonary hypertension (PH) is alleviated [3], but there is no proof that this may occur in humans. While microvascular disease has been labeled as the target for medical treatments of CTEPH [4], major vessel lesions are the target for PEA and BPA, with excellent outcomes.

CTEPH is curable by PEA which comprises a mechanical entry into a thrombus plane in the proximal pulmonary artery and removal of a dissectate that represents the inside of the pulmonary arterial tree. However, about 40–50% of

© Springer Nature Switzerland AG 2022
F. Saia et al. (eds.), *Balloon pulmonary angioplasty in patients with CTEPH*,
https://doi.org/10.1007/978-3-030-95997-5_6

patients are not eligible for surgery due to distal lesions or due to comorbidities resulting in an unfavorable risk/benefit ratio for PEA. In addition, 17–51% of patients experience persistent or recurrent PH after PEA [5] [6] [7] [8]. In a majority, these cases are candidates for BPA which is an emerging percutaneous method that effectively restores flow in narrowed or completely obstructed pulmonary arteries of patients with inoperable CTEPH or persistent PH after PEA. In contrast to PEA, BPA targets lesions focally, oftentimes at the bifurcations. The mechanism of BPA is the fracture of intravascular webs and bands [9] or controlled perforation of collagen plugs in the case of total occlusions restoring flow to dependent vascular territories. In contrast to percutaneous coronary angioplasty, BPA does not injure the medial layer of the vessel, and therefore in-lesion restenosis does not occur [10]. Lesions have been classified [11] into (type A) ring-like stenoses, (type B) web lesions, (type C) subtotal occlusions, (type D) chronic total occlusions, and (type E) tortuous lesions.

The exclusivity of PEA because of few surgeons in the world, complexity of the procedure, and challenging logistics leaving more than 50% of cases untreated has been a driver for alternative treatments. While medical treatment (reviewed in Chap. 4) has rapidly recruited patients in randomized controlled trials (RCT) and been successfully approved for the treatment of not-operable CTEPH or persistent-recurrent PH after PEA [12, 13], BPA was first performed in 1988 in Europe [14], but was then abandoned because of a high complication rate in an initial US series [15]. Over the past two decades the technique was refined by Japanese operators [16–19] and has since then reentered Europe [20–23, 24]. It has to be kept in mind that randomized controlled trials (RCTs) testing the relative efficacy and safety of BPA against PEA are missing at this time. Observational registries demonstrated that 6-minute walking distance (6-MWD) improvement is significantly greater after BPA than after medical therapy for CTEPH ($p = 0.001$)

[25]. A single RCT testing the efficacy and safety of BPA against medical therapy with riociguat has reported 26-week data in fall 2019 (RACE trial NCT02634203), but has remained unpublished. By week 26, geometric mean PVR decreased to 41% of baseline value in 52 patients of the BPA group, compared with 68% of baseline value in 53 patients of the riociguat group. While these data suggest greater efficacy of BPA, complication rates were higher in patients undergoing BPA.

In this chapter current clinical outcomes of BPA based on observational studies will be summarized with regard to hemodynamic changes, changes in the World Health Organization functional class (WHO FC), 6-MWD, and complications (Table 6.1). The data show that BPA results in marked improvements in pulmonary hemodynamics and exercise capacity indicating its efficacy and safety. Further endpoints such as quality of life, effect on right ventricular function (RVF), and cardiopulmonary exercise testing will be reported from smaller series.

6.2   Indications for BPA

BPA is indicated in patients with CTEPH who have comorbidities precluding surgery and are technically inoperable, e.g., due to predominantly distal lesions [29], patient preference, and a lack of clinical expertise for PEA, and in the preoperative setting of high-risk CTEPH patients undergoing noncardiac surgeries [30]. In a recent series of inoperable CTEPH patients, baseline New York Heart Association functional class, right atrial pressure (RAP), and 6-min walk distance (6-MWD) were found as independent predictors of survival. Multivariate analysis found that baseline 6-MWD (per 20 m increase in distance) (hazard ratio [HR], 0.879; 95% confidence interval [CI], 0.832–0.928, $p < 0.001$) and BPA (HR, 0.307; 95% CI, 0.099–0.957; $p = 0.042$) were independently associated with survival [31], underscoring the importance of BPA in this population.

Table 6.1 Clinical outcomes of BPA in published series with ≥50 treated patients, including the first European and the first US series for comparison

	French reference centre [24]	Hannover and Bad Nauheim [22]	Japanese Multicenter Registry led by Okayama [26]	Sendai series [27]	Tokyo series [28]	Oslo series [20]	First US series [15]
	184	56	308	84	170	20	18
Age (years)	63 ± 14	65 (55–74)	62 ± 13	65 +/− 14	66 years (25th and 75th percentiles, 55 and 73 years)	60 ± 10	Mean age, 51.8; range, 14–75
Female (%)	49	61	80	81	78	50	Not stated
Number of procedures	1006	266	1408	424	649	371	47
Procedure number/person	5 (median)	5 (median)	4 (median)	5.0 ± 2.5	4 (median)	3.7 ± 2.1 (2–9)	2.6 (1–5)
Technical details	0.014-inch wires	0.014-inch wires	Predominantly 0.014-inch wires, CTOs are treated	3D reconstructed computed tomography guidance, and OCT	None specified	Direct guiding catheter engagement, mainly 0.014-inch wires	0.035-inch wires, guide catheter was a 7-French high-flow pigtail where most of the curled tip was removed

	French [24] Baseline	French [24] After BPA	Hannover [22] Baseline	Hannover [22] After BPA	Japanese [26] Baseline	Japanese [26] After BPA	Sendai [27] Baseline	Sendai [27] After BPA	Tokyo [28] Baseline	Tokyo [28] After BPA	Oslo [20] Baseline	Oslo [20] After BPA	US [15] Baseline	US [15] After BPA
Patient number	154		56	55	308	196	77		170	170	20		18	
Repeat evaluation (months after last BPA)	3–6		6		12.2 ± 13.3		6		6–18 (short term)		3		1–40	
6-MWD (m)	396 ± 120	441 ± 104	358 ± 108	391 ± 108	318 ± 122	430 ± 109	380 ± 138	486 ± 112	Not stated	Not stated	CPET instead	CPET instead	191	454.5
WHO I&II vs. III&IV	35.3/64.7	78.7/21.3	15.0/85.0	73.0/25.0	Median 3	Median 2	68.0/28.0	Not stated	Not stated	Not stated	3.0 ± 0.5	2.0 ± 0.5	3.3	1.8
mPAP (mmHg)	43.9 ± 9.5	31.6 ± 9.0	40 ± 12	33 ± 11	43.2 ± 11.0	22.5 ± 5.4	38 ± 10	25 ± 6	38*	22*	45 ± 11	33 ± 10	43 ± 12.1	33.7 ± 10.2
paO2 (mmHg)	65.0 ± 9.0	73.3 ± 12.0	62.0 ± 9.0	66.0 ± 10.0	Not stated	Not stated	Not stated	Not stated	Not stated	Not stated	Not stated	Not stated	Not stated	Not stated
SaO2 (%)	Not stated	Not stated	93.0 ± 3.0	94.0 ± 3.0	93.3 ± 4.5	94.0 ± 5.2	87.5 ± 5.3	91.9 ± 4.3	Not stated	Not stated	90 ± 5	93 ± 4	Not stated	Not stated
Peak VO2, mL/kg/min	Not done	Not done	Not done	Not done	Not done	Not done	Not done	Not done	Not stated	Not stated	13.6 ± 5.6	17.0 ± 6.5	Not stated	Not stated
CO (L/min)	4.8 ± 1.2	5.6 ± 1.4	4.4 ± 1.1	4.6 ± 1.2	Not stated	Not stated	Not stated	Not stated	Not stated	Not stated	4.9 ± 1.6	5.4 ± 1.9	Not stated	Not stated

(continued)

Table 6.1 (continued)

	French reference centre [24]		Hannover and Bad Nauheim [22]		Japanese Multicenter Registry led by Okayama [26]		Sendai series [27]		Tokyo series [28]		Oslo series [20]		First US series [15]	
CI (L/min/m²)	2.7 ± 0.6	3.1 ± 0.8	2.4 ± 0.6	2.5 ± 0.6	2.6 ± 0.8	2.8 ± 0.6	2.7 ± 0.7	2.5 ± 0.5	2.6*	3.1*	Not stated	Not stated	2.0 ± 0 0.4	2.1 ± 0 0.6
PVR (dyne · s · cm⁻⁵)	604 ± 226	329 ± 177	591 ± 286	440 ± 279	854 ± 450	288 ± 195	584 ± 256	304 ± 80	600 *	200 *	704 ± 320	472 ± 288	TPR: 1832 ± 720	TPR: 1360 ± 640
Patients (%) on riociguat and/or drugs approved for PAH	62	Not stated	92	Not stated	72	45	96	68 chronic 41	91,2	40.8	10	Not stated	No medications approved back then, off-label not stated	
Lung injury (% of sessions)	9.1		9.4		17.8		8		Not stated		35		23	
30-day mortality (%)	2.2		1.8		2.6		0		2.3		10		5.5	

Data taken from illustration as in [28].

6-MWD = 6-min walking distance, *BPA* = balloon pulmonary angioplasty, *CO* = cardiac output, *CI* = cardiac index, *CTEPH* = chronic thromboembolic pulmonary hypertension, *mPAP* = mean pulmonary artery pressure, *PEA* = pulmonary endarterectomy, *peak VO2* = peak oxygen consumption, *PVR* = pulmonary vascular resistance; *SaO2* = arterial oxygen saturation, *WHO* = World Health Organization;

6.3 Effect of BPA on Hemodynamics

Mechanical treatments of CTEPH, i.e., PEA and BPA, have conferred substantial improvement of hemodynamics that are beyond any changes obtained with vasodilator treatments of non-vasoreactive subjects with precapillary non-thromboembolic PH. In contrast to PEA, BPA constitutes a series of procedures [4–20] upsizing balloons to gradually decrease pressures. BPA does not produce immediate hemodynamic improvement at the time of the procedure, but only after some time. Therefore, operators have agreed to report hemodynamic data at baseline immediately before the first BPA, and to report final data 3–6 months after the final BPA. Complete treatment of a lesion may be formally defined as pulmonary flow grade 3 [32], a ratio of distal:proximal pressures across the target lesion (detected by pressure wire) >0.8, and mean pulmonary arterial pressure distal to a treated lesion <35 mmHg (as determined by pressure wire without vasodilation) [32]. "Complete BPA" is defined as complete treatment of all identifiable and accessible lesions, and/or when the hemodynamic target has been reached. Targets still differ, some groups targeting pressures below the definition of normal [33], and the practice of adding vasodilator treatments to BPA treatments varies, but vasodilator treatments do factor-in the hemodynamic response [34]. It is important to note that vasodilator treatments mainly affect cardiac output (CO) [12, 13, 34, 35], while BPA also affects mean pulmonary artery pressure (mPAP) [22, 24, 26].

Table 6.1 illustrates short-term result of BPA [26]. Long-term results were maintained at 50.3 months [28], and appear to be sustained up to 10 years with 89.7% survival (unpublished data on 414 patients).

In 2017, the first multicenter registry of patients undergoing BPA at seven Japanese institutions demonstrated substantial improvements in hemodynamics at a relatively low complication rate [26]. In the same year the first German experience was published from the Hannover and Bad Nauheim centers [22] (Table 6.1). In 2019

the French reference centers published the results from 184 inoperable CTEPH patients who underwent 1006 BPA sessions. While the Japanese multicenter registry reported a postprocedural mPAP of 22 mmHg, postprocedural mPAP in the French dataset was of 31 mmHg (Table 6.1), with baseline mPAP of 43 mmHg in both datasets [36]. While the exact timing of follow-up catheterization may account for some of the variation, differences in post-BPA vasodilator treatments and operator experience may play a role. However, published data suggest that there are intrinsic differences in metabolic and coagulation markers between Japanese and European CTEPH [4, 37]. Another of those differences is the change of CO with BPA. While European patients experience improvement, Japanese patients undergoing BPA hardly change CO and cardiac index. These observations may signify an ethnology-dependent characteristic of RV remodeling, potentially in association with RV fibrosis [38]. Despite the greater effect on CO in European patients, decrease of pulmonary vascular resistance (PVR) was significantly greater in Japanese patients (Table 6.1).

A small Polish series documented favorable effects of BPA in 10 patients with a median age of 81 [75–88] with a 6-MWD distance increased from a median of 221 m (80–320) to 345 m (230–455) (P < 0.01). No severe complications occurred during BPA and over a median follow-up of 553 days (range 81–784) [21]. The multicentric Polish BPA registry will soon report national data. Another series reporting favorable results in ≥70-year-olds comes from Japan [29]. Today, BPA is spreading all over the world [39–43] [44] and is being used for any condition that results in CTEPH [45].

Several meta-analyses and reviews further support the beneficial effects of BPA on pulmonary hemodynamics. Tanabe et al. reviewed 26 non-randomized studies in 2018 of which 13 studies (493 patients) were selected: the 10 most recent ones including complete data from each institution [46]. Mean pulmonary arterial pressure decreased from 39.4–56 to 20.9–36 mmHg, and the 6-min walk distance increased from 191–405 to 359–501 m. 2-year mortality of

80 patients undergoing BPA was significantly lower compared to 68 patients receiving only medical treatment (1.3% vs. 13.2%); the risk ratio was 0.14 (95% confidence interval: 0.03–0.76).

In a meta-analysis by Zoppellaro et al., 14 studies were included (725 patients), showing that BPA was associated with a reduction in mean pulmonary artery pressure (from 43 to 32.5 mmHg), reduction in pulmonary vascular resistance (from 9.94 to 5.06 wood units), increase in cardiac index (from 2.35 to 2.62 L/min/m^2), and improvement of 6-minute walking distance (from 345 to 442 m) [47].

In a second meta-analysis [48], BPA resulted in significantly decreased mean pulmonary artery pressure (−14.2 mmHg [95% CI -18.9, −9.5]), PVR (−303.5 dyn.s/cm [5] [95% CI -377.6, −229.4]), and mean RAP (−2.7 mmHg [95% CI -4.1, −1.3]) in 17 noncomparative studies comprising 670 CTEPH patients (mean age 62 years; 68% women). 6-MWD (67.3 m [95% CI 53.8, 80.8]) and CO (0.2 l/min [95% CI 0.0, 0.3]) increased after BPA.

6.4 Effect of BPA on WHO Functional Class, Cardiopulmonary Exercise Capacity, and Respiratory Function

Better cardiopulmonary function was observed in patients with CTEPH after BPA, paralleling hemodynamic improvement [49, 50]. Percent predicted diffusion capacity for carbon monoxide (DLCO) decreased after BPA in the lower lung field but the ventilation/CO2 production (V˙e/V˙CO2) slope significantly improved after BPA in the lower lobes [51]. However, in a recent abstract at the European Society of Cardiology Meeting 2020 Matsuyoka et al. from Kobe reported that while BPA could dramatically improve hemodynamics and exercise tolerance, arterial oxygenation was not normalized after BPA. Oxygen desaturation under exercise, and diffusing capacity for carbon monoxide (%DLCO/VA), remained unchanged in their series. Arterial oxygenation has been found to be the last parameter to improve during BPA treatments. In the Tokyo series [28], freedom from home oxygen therapy was 15.3% at baseline, 29.0% (95% CI, 17.2–41.8) at midterm, and 38.6% (95% CI, 25.0–52.0) at long-term follow-up after BPA.

6.5 Effect of BPA on Right Ventricular Function

BPA improves RV function by alleviating RV dyssynchrony [52]. This observation was confirmed by a study where RV electromechanical delay and dispersion by speckle tracking echocardiography significantly improved after BPA [53]. For LV and RV free walls, the time to peak (Tpeak) of circumferential strain was calculated by cardiac magnetic resonance as a parameter for interventricular dyssynchrony. Increased left ventricular end-diastolic volume ($r = 0.65$, $p < 0.01$), SV ($r = 0.74$, $p < 0.001$), and 6-MWD ($r = 0.54$, $p < 0.05$) were correlated to the reduction in left-right delay [54].

6.6 Effect of BPA on Quality of Life (QoL)

Twenty-five patients with inoperable or persistent CTEPH filled out the 36-item Short Form (SF-36v2) questionnaire prior to BPA treatment and after ≥3 BPA sessions. The mental component summary score of QoL improved after completion of treatment in parallel with improvement in 6-MWD [23].

In the UK series [44], 30 consecutive, inoperable, anatomically suitable, symptomatic patients undergoing one to six BPA sessions reduced their QoL (CAMPHOR symptom score: 8.7 ± 5.4 vs. 5.6 ± 6.1, $p = 0.0005$) in parallel with reductions in pulmonary pressures (mean PAP: 44.7 ± 11.0 vs. 34.4 ± 8.3 mm Hg, $p < 0.0001$), PVR ($663 ± 281$ vs. $436 ± 196$ dyn.s.cm^{-5}, $p < 0.0001$), WHO functional class, and exercise capacity (6-MWD: $366 ± 107$ vs. $440 ± 94$ m, $p < 0.0001$).

6.7   Effect of BPA on Survival

Survival data derived from large registries (Table 6.1) report data that exceed survival of pulmonary arterial hypertension (PAH). For example, in the French registry 3-year survival was 95.1% [24], and in the Japanese multicenter registry 94.5% (95% confidence interval, 89.3–97.3%) [26]. In Tanabe's review no significant difference was observed in the 2-year mortality between BPA (n = 97) and PEA ($n = 63$) patients [46]. From 12 studies reporting mortality with median follow-up of 9 months after BPA (range, 1–51 months) [48], pooled incidence of short (≤ 1 month) and greater than one-month mortality was 1.9% and 5.7%, respectively.

6.8   Effects of BPA on Renal Function

BPA not only improves pulmonary but also affects systemic hemodynamics. 51 patients undergoing 5 (±2) BPA sessions received 133 (±48; 21–300) mL of contrast agent per session and 691 (±24; 240–1410) mL during the entire treatment series. Acute kidney injury occurred after 6 (2.3%) procedures. Creatinine [80.1 (IQR 67.8–96.8) μmol/L vs. 77.4 (IQR 66.9–91.5) μmol/L, $p = 0.02$] and urea level [13.7 (IQR10.7–16.6) mmol/L vs. 12.5 (IQR 10.0–15.5) mmol/L, $p = 0.02$] decreased from baseline to the 6-month follow-up. Estimated glomerular filtration rate (eGFR) [79 (IQR 59–94) mL/min/m^2 vs. 79.6 (IQR 67.1–95.0) mL/min/m^2, $p = 0.11$] did not change. In patients with chronic kidney disease stage ≥ 2 an increase of eGFR occurred, and a decrease of creatinine and urea from baseline to 6-month follow-up. BPA

improves pulmonary and systemic hemodynamics, with positive effects on renal function. Repetitive administration of contrast agent in expert hands does not appear to be harmful regarding renal function [55].

In the Polish experience, GFR did not change significantly within 72 h after BPA. Significant improvement was noted in GFR (75.4 ± 21.2 vs. 80.9 ± 22.4 mL/min/1.73 m^2; $p = 0.012$) in addition to improvement in RAP (9.1 ± 4.1 to 5.0 ± 2.2 mm Hg; $p < 0.001$), mean PAP (49.1 ± 10.7 to 29.8 ± 8.3 mm Hg; $p < 0.001$), CI (CI; 2.42 ± 0.6 to 2.70 ± 0.6 L/min/m^2; $p = 0.004$), and PVR (9.42 ± 3.6 to 4.4 ± 2.3 wood units; $p < 0.001$). In 12 patients with impaired renal function at baseline, relative increase in GFR was significantly correlated with relative improvement in CI ($r = 0.060$; $p = 0.037$), RAP ($r = -0.587$; $p = 0.044$), and mixed venous saturation ($r = 0.069$; $p = 0.012$) [56].

6.9   BPA in Specific Situations (Table 6.2)

Two studies have reported rescue BPA after unsuccessful PEA [57, 58]. While one of the strengths of percutaneous intervention is its rapid availability, BPA does not immediately relieve pressures, but needs extracorporeal membrane oxygenation (ECMO) support. Simultaneous PEA and BPA have raised considerable interest particularly as BPA can be performed under the protection of cardiopulmonary bypass under low pulmonary pressure conditions, but this technique has remained confined to the Bad Nauheim center [59].

BPA is also efficiently changing hemodynamics in chronic thromboembolic disease (CTED) [64, 65]. In the German CTED series PVR decreased from 234 ± 68 dyne · s · cm^{-5} to 167 ± 40 dyne · s · cm^{-5}, at the cost of one case of mild hemoptysis [65]. While Wiedenroth's patients were not operable, a UK series of PEA in CTED was performed. PEA in these patients

Table 6.2 Clinical outcomes of BPA performed as rescue after PEA, simultaneous with PEA or elective after PEA, in published series

	Rescue after PEA		Simultaneous with PEA	Elective after PEA			
	Nakamura et al. [57]	Collaud et al. [58]	German series [59]	Leuven experience [60]	Polish series [61]	Kobe series [62]	Tokyo series [63]
Total patient number	1	3	3	18 (5 after PEA)	15	44	9
Age (y)	41	65.3	65.3 ± 6.4	61 ± 19	50.4 ± 13.5	63.9 ± 2.5	55.1 (44.9–61.7)
Female (%)	100	66	1 (33)	55	40	9 (90)	77
Number of procedures	1	1	3	91	71	24	44
Procedure number/person	1	1	1	4 (2–8)	4.7 ± 1.4	2.4 ± 0.3	Not stated
Time between the PEA and the first BPA session	6 days	POD 16, POD 3, POD 1	0	Not stated	28.1 ± 25.8 months	7.3 ± 2.3 months	49.2 (32.4–94.8) months
(hemodynamic timing)			Baseline / After PEA/BPA	Before / After BPA	Baseline / After PEA and BPA	Baseline / After PEA and BPA	After BPA / After PEA and BPA
Patient number	1	3	3	18 (post-PEA not separately reported)	15	44 (10 after PEA with BPA)	9
Repeat hemodynamic evaluation after last BPA	Na	One survivor POD24	Postoperative day 1	72 days (range, 26–282 days)	1–1.5 months	6 months	22.8 (15.6–39.6) months
6-MWD (m)	Na		Not stated	412 ± 167 / 402 ± 196	383 ± 104 / 476 ± 107	338 ± 62 / 429 ± 38	358 ± 108 / 391 ± 108
WHO	Na		3.6 ± 0.6 / 1.3 ± 0.6	2 (1–4) / 2 (1–3)	1 patient class IV, 8 class III, and 6 class II / 2 patients class III, 11 class II, and 2 class I	0/5/4/1 / 7/3/0/0	3 patients class II, 5 class III, 1 class IV / 7 patients class I, 2 class II
mPAP (mmHg)	50 / 23	58	64.6 ± 0.6 / 37.6 ± 7.5	44 ± 12 / 31 ± 12	44.7 ± 6.4 / 30.8 ± 7.5	26.9 ± 3.1 / 18.7 ± 1.7	43 (30–52) / 26 (21–29)
SaO$_2$ (%)	Not stated		Not stated	Not stated / Not stated	95 ± 2.3 / 95.25 ± 4.5	95.6 ± 0.7 / 94.0 ± 0.6	Not stated / Not available
Peak VO2, mL/kg/min	Na		Na	Not stated / Not stated	Not stated / Not stated	15.0 ± 2.1 / 17.7 ± 1.8	Not available
CO (L/min)	5.5	4.6	Not stated	4.3 ± 1.0 / 5.0 ± 1.1*	5.34 ± 1.4 / 5.27 ± 1.23	Not stated	3.9 (3.4–4.3) / 4.2 (3.2–4.8)

CI (L/min/m^2)	4.0	Not stated		2.3 ± 0.4	2.7 ± 0.6	2.9 ± 0.74	2.9 ± 0.9	2.2 ± 0.2	2.3 ± 0.2	Not stated	Not stated
PVR (dyne · s · cm^{-5})	340 / 1170	1360 ± 440.8	518.6 ± 146,1	672 ± 288	368 ± 264	551.9 ± 185.2	343.8 ± 123.8	386 ± 42	244 ± 35	648 (488–984)	320 (224–384)
Patients (%) on riociguat and/or drugs approved for PAH	100	100	Not stated	72	Not stated	100	86	40	Not stated	Not stated	Not stated
Lung injury (% of sessions)	100	100		5.4		2.8		33.3		2.3	
30-day mortality (%)	0 / 66	0		0		0		0		0	

na = not applicable, *6-MWD* = 6-min walking distance, *BPA* = balloon pulmonary angioplasty, *CO* = cardiac output, *CI* = cardiac index, *CTEPH* = chronic thromboembolic pulmonary hypertension, *mPAP* = mean pulmonary artery pressure, *PEA* = pulmonary endarterectomy, *peak VO2* = peak oxygen consumption, *PVR* = pulmonary vascular resistance, *SaO2* = arterial oxygen saturation, *WHO* = World Health Organization.

resulted in no in-hospital mortality but in a 40% complication rate [66], predominantly supraventricular arrhythmias requiring cardioversion or wound problems. MPAP (21 ± 5 mmHg to 18 ± 5 mmHg) and PVR (164 ± 104 mmHg to 128 ± 60 mmHg) decreased significantly.

6.10 Complications

Table 6.1 summarizes complication rates after BPA. Vascular injury is a major cause of lung injury after BPA in patients with CTEPH [67]. In contrast, reperfusion pulmonary edema is much rarer, and occurs late, after 24–72 hours. In line with data that are shown in Table 6.1, Tanabe's review [46] showed an early mortality of BPA between 0% and 14.3%; lung injury occurred in 7.0% to 31.4% of sessions. In a multivariate analysis of 873 lesions, occlusive lesions were the sole independent predictor of procedure-related complications (adjusted odds ratio 5.83, 95% CI [1.94–17.47], $p = 0.002$). Baseline hemodynamic was not a predictor of complications [68]. However, in the French series per-patient multivariate analysis revealed that baseline mPAP (odds ratio [OR], 1.08; 95% [CI], 1.039 1.130; $p < 0.001$) and the period during which BPA procedure was performed (recent versus initial period; OR, 0.367; 95% CI, 0.175–0.771; $p = 0.008$) were significant factors related to lung injury. In Zoppellaro's meta-analysis [47] periprocedural deaths occurred in 2.1% of patients (95% CI 0.8–4.1) while reperfusion and pulmonary vessel injuries were reported in 9.3% (95% CI 3.1–18.4) and 2.3% (95% CI 0.9–4.5) of sessions, respectively. All series are reporting learning curves, with significantly less complications over time [24], including shortening of hospital stays after BPA [69].

6.11 Clinical Limitations of BPA

Current conventional indication for BPA is surgically inoperability [41], and textbook literature [70] points out that subsegmental and distal diseases are primary targets for BPA. However, in the learning curve of BPA in many centers it has become clear that excellent results of BPA are achieved in the lobar and segmental vessels that have been the primary targets for PEA. Very distal arteries, i.e., ≤2 mm in cross-sectional diameter, that cannot be reached by the finest surgical equipment are usually also no good targets for BPA. According to the lesion classification of Kawakami et al. [11], chronic total occlusions, particularly type D lesions, are important targets, but oftentimes hard to open, and commonly lead to complications. One further limitation of BPA is that the number of lesions is oftentimes hard to handle for single operators or operator pairs, and requires repeated sessions. Radiation and contrast are clear limitations in these settings. Subsets of CTEPH with severe microvascular disease components, e.g., patients after splenectomy, pose particular challenges. Taniguchi and colleagues reported that poor subpleural perfusion, suggesting the presence of microvascular disease, can be observed in 15% of the patients and is associated with decreased response to BPA treatment [2].

Finally, comorbidities in the CTEPH population aggravate procedural burden on patients, e.g., old age, neurologic disease, malignancy, chronic pain, depression, and irreversible pulmonary parenchymal damage. Persistently impaired oxygenation due to residual high intrapulmonary shunt fraction after BPA remains associated with reduced exercise tolerance [71].

6.12 Discussion and Conclusion

Recent data have confirmed the overall clinical safety and efficacy of BPA for the treatment of inoperable CTEPH and persistent/recurrent PH. We have learned that the absolute change in mPAP was directly related to the number of treated segments [17], impacting WHO functional class, 6-MWD, and quality of life. The clinical effect of BPA is sustained, and in many CTEPH centers in Europe observational data suggest that the effect of BPA is similar to PEA. In CTEPH centers, BPA is likely to be no stand-alone treatment strategy, but used in complementarity with PEA and medical therapies.

Acknowledgment This research was funded by the Austrian Science Fund F54.

Disclosure IML has relationships with drug companies including AOP Orphan Pharmaceuticals AG, Actelion-Janssen, MSD, Medtronic, and Ferrer. In addition to being an investigator in trials involving these companies, relationships include consultancy service, research grants, and membership of scientific advisory boards.

References

1. Gerges C, Gerges M, Friewald R, Fesler P, Dorfmuller P, Sharma S, et al. Microvascular disease in chronic thromboembolic pulmonary hypertension: hemodynamic phenotyping and Histomorphometric assessment. Circulation. 2020;141(5):376–86.
2. Taniguchi Y, Brenot P, Jais X, Garcia C, Weatherald J, Planche O, et al. Poor subpleural perfusion predicts failure after balloon pulmonary angioplasty for non-operable chronic thromboembolic pulmonary hypertension. Chest. 2018;154(3):521–31.
3. Boulate D, Perros F, Dorfmuller P, Arthur-Ataam J, Guihaire J, Lamrani L, et al. Pulmonary microvascular lesions regress in reperfused chronic thromboembolic pulmonary hypertension. J Heart Lung Transplant. 2015;34(3):457–67.
4. Lang IM, Madani M. Update on chronic thromboembolic pulmonary hypertension. Circulation. 2014;130(6):508–18.
5. Pepke-Zaba J, Delcroix M, Lang I, Mayer E, Jansa P, Ambroz D, et al. Chronic thromboembolic pulmonary hypertension (CTEPH): results from an international prospective registry. Circulation. 2011;124(18):1973–81.
6. Archibald CJ, Auger WR, Fedullo PF, Channick RN, Kerr KM, Jamieson SW, et al. Long-term outcome after pulmonary thromboendarterectomy. Am J Respir Crit Care Med. 1999;160(2):523–8.
7. Skoro-Sajer N, Marta G, Gerges C, Hlavin G, Nierlich P, Taghavi S, et al. Surgical specimens, haemodynamics and long-term outcomes after pulmonary endarterectomy. Thorax. 2014;69(2):116–22.
8. Cannon JE, Su L, Kiely DG, Page K, Toshner M, Swietlik E, et al. Dynamic risk stratification of patient long-term outcome after pulmonary endarterectomy: results from the United Kingdom National Cohort. Circulation. 2016;133(18):1761–71.
9. Räber L, Ueki Y, Lang IM. Balloon pulmonary angioplasty for the treatment of chronic thromboembolic pulmonary hypertension. EuroIntervention. 2019;15(9):e814–5.
10. Lang I, Meyer BC, Ogo T, Matsubara H, Kurzyna M, Ghofrani HA, et al. Balloon pulmonary angioplasty in chronic thromboembolic pulmonary hypertension. European respiratory review: an official journal of the European respiratory. Society. 2017;26:143.
11. Kawakami T, Ogawa A, Miyaji K, Mizoguchi H, Shimokawahara H, Naito T, et al. Novel angiographic classification of each vascular lesion in chronic thromboembolic pulmonary hypertension based on selective angiogram and results of balloon pulmonary angioplasty. Circ Cardiovasc Interv. 2016;9:10.
12. Ghofrani HA, D'Armini AM, Grimminger F, Hoeper MM, Jansa P, Kim NH, et al. Riociguat for the treatment of chronic thromboembolic pulmonary hypertension. N Engl J Med. 2013;369(4):319–29.
13. Sadushi-Kolici R, Jansa P, Kopec G, Torbicki A, Skoro-Sajer N, Campean IA, et al. Subcutaneous treprostinil for the treatment of severe non-operable chronic thromboembolic pulmonary hypertension (CTREPH): a double-blind, phase 3, randomised controlled trial. Lancet Respir Med. 2019;7(3):239–48.
14. Voorburg JA, Cats VM, Buis B, Bruschke AV. Balloon angioplasty in the treatment of pulmonary hypertension caused by pulmonary embolism. Chest. 1988;94(6):1249–53.
15. Feinstein JA, Goldhaber SZ, Lock JE, Ferndandes SM, Landzberg MJ. Balloon pulmonary angioplasty for treatment of chronic thromboembolic pulmonary hypertension. Circulation. 2001;103(1):10–3.
16. Kataoka M, Inami T, Hayashida K, Shimura N, Ishiguro H, Abe T, et al. Percutaneous transluminal pulmonary angioplasty for the treatment of chronic thromboembolic pulmonary hypertension. Circ Cardiovasc Interv. 2012;5(6):756–62.
17. Mizoguchi H, Ogawa A, Munemasa M, Mikouchi H, Ito H, Matsubara H. Refined balloon pulmonary angioplasty for inoperable patients with chronic thromboembolic pulmonary hypertension. Circ Cardiovasc Interv. 2012;5(6):748–55.
18. Sugimura K, Fukumoto Y, Satoh K, Nochioka K, Miura Y, Aoki T, et al. Percutaneous transluminal pulmonary angioplasty markedly improves pulmonary hemodynamics and long-term prognosis in patients with chronic thromboembolic pulmonary hypertension. Circ J. 2012;76(2):485–8.
19. Taniguchi Y, Miyagawa K, Nakayama K, Kinutani H, Shinke T, Okada K, et al. Balloon pulmonary angioplasty: an additional treatment option to improve the prognosis of patients with chronic thromboembolic pulmonary hypertension. EuroIntervention. 2014;10(4):518–25.
20. Andreassen AK, Ragnarsson A, Gude E, Geiran O, Andersen R. Balloon pulmonary angioplasty in patients with inoperable chronic thromboembolic pulmonary hypertension. Heart. 2013;99(19):1415–20.
21. Roik M, Wretowski D, Łabyk A, Irzyk K, Lichodziejewska B, Dzikowska-Diduch O, et al. Refined balloon pulmonary angioplasty-a therapeutic option in very elderly patients with chronic thromboembolic pulmonary hypertension. J Interv Cardiol. 2017;30(3):249–55.
22. Olsson KM, Wiedenroth CB, Kamp JC, Breithecker A, Fuge J, Krombach GA, et al. Balloon pulmonary angioplasty for inoperable patients with chronic

thromboembolic pulmonary hypertension: the initial German experience. Eur Respir J. 2017;49:6.

23. Darocha S, Pietura R, Pietrasik A, Norwa J, Dobosiewicz A, Pilka M, et al. Improvement in quality of life and hemodynamics in chronic thromboembolic pulmonary hypertension treated with balloon pulmonary angioplasty. Circulation. 2017;81(4):552–7.

24. Brenot P, Jais X, Taniguchi Y, Garcia Alonso C, Gerardin B, Mussot S, et al. French experience of balloon pulmonary angioplasty for chronic thromboembolic pulmonary hypertension. Eur Respir J. 2019;53:5.

25. Phan K, Jo HE, Xu J, Lau EM. Medical therapy versus balloon angioplasty for CTEPH: a systematic review and meta-analysis. Heart Lung Circ. 2018;27(1):89–98.

26. Ogawa A, Satoh T, Fukuda T, Sugimura K, Fukumoto Y, Emoto N, et al. Balloon pulmonary angioplasty for chronic thromboembolic pulmonary hypertension: results of a multicenter registry. Circ Cardiovasc Qual Outcomes. 2017;10:11.

27. Aoki T, Sugimura K, Tatebe S, Miura M, Yamamoto S, Yaoita N, et al. Comprehensive evaluation of the effectiveness and safety of balloon pulmonary angioplasty for inoperable chronic thrombo-embolic pulmonary hypertension: long-term effects and procedure-related complications. Eur Heart J. 2017;38(42):3152–9.

28. Inami T, Kataoka M, Yanagisawa R, Ishiguro H, Shimura N, Fukuda K, et al. Long-term outcomes after percutaneous transluminal pulmonary angioplasty for chronic thromboembolic pulmonary hypertension. Circulation. 2016;134(24):2030–2.

29. Yamagata Y, Ikeda S, Nakata T, Yonekura T, Koga S, Muroya T, et al. Balloon pulmonary angioplasty is effective for treating peripheral-type chronic thromboembolic pulmonary hypertension in elderly patients. Geriatr Gerontol Int. 2018;18(5):678–84.

30. Watanabe K, Ito N, Ohata T, Kariya T, Inui H, Yamada Y. Preoperative balloon pulmonary angioplasty enabled noncardiac surgery of a patient with chronic thromboembolic pulmonary hypertension (CTEPH): a case report. Medicine. 2019;98(10):e14807.

31. Taniguchi Y, Jaïs X, Jevnikar M, Boucly A, Weatherald J, Brenot P, et al. Predictors of survival in patients with not-operated chronic thromboembolic pulmonary hypertension. J Heart Lung Transplant. 2019;38(8):833–42.

32. Inami T, Kataoka M, Shimura N, Ishiguro H, Yanagisawa R, Taguchi H, et al. Pulmonary edema predictive scoring index (PEPSI), a new index to predict risk of reperfusion pulmonary edema and improvement of hemodynamics in percutaneous transluminal pulmonary angioplasty. JACC Cardiovasc Interv. 2013;6(7):725–36.

33. Shinkura Y, Nakayama K, Yanaka K, Kinutani H, Tamada N, Tsuboi Y, et al. Extensive revascularisation by balloon pulmonary angioplasty for chronic thromboembolic pulmonary hypertension beyond haemodynamic normalisation. EuroIntervention. 2018;13(17):2060–8.

34. Wiedenroth CB, Ghofrani HA, Adameit MSD, Breithecker A, Haas M, Kriechbaum S, et al. Sequential treatment with riociguat and balloon pulmonary angioplasty for patients with inoperable chronic thromboembolic pulmonary hypertension. Pulmonary Circulation. 2018;8(3):2045894018783996.

35. Wang W, Wen L, Song Z, Shi W, Wang K, Huang W. Balloon pulmonary angioplasty vs riociguat in patients with inoperable chronic thromboembolic pulmonary hypertension: a systematic review and meta-analysis. Clin Cardiol. 2019;42(8):741–52.

36. Lang IM, Matsubara H. Balloon pulmonary angioplasty for the treatment of chronic thromboembolic pulmonary hypertension: is Europe behind? Eur Respir J. 2019;53:1900843.

37. Chausheva S, Naito A, Ogawa A, Seidl V, Winter MP, Sharma S, et al. Chronic thromboembolic pulmonary hypertension in Austria and Japan. J Thorac Cardiovasc Surg. 2019;158(2):604–14.

38. Ozawa K, Funabashi N, Takaoka H, Tanabe N, Tatsumi K, Kobayashi Y. Detection of right ventricular myocardial fibrosis using quantitative CT attenuation of the right ventricular myocardium in the late phase on 320 slice CT in subjects with pulmonary hypertension. Int J Cardiol. 2017;228:165–8.

39. Velázquez Martín M, Albarrán González-Trevilla A, Alonso Charterina S, García Tejada J, Cortina Romero JM, Escribano SP. Balloon pulmonary angioplasty for inoperable patients with chronic thromboembolic pulmonary hypertension. Preliminary experience in Spain in a series of 7 patients. Rev Esp Cardiol. 2015;68(6):535–7.

40. de Waard GA, Melenhorst MC, van Leeuwen MA, Bogaard HJ, Lely RJ, van Royen N. Balloon pulmonary angioplasty for chronic thromboembolic pulmonary hypertension. Ned Tijdschr Geneeskd. 2016;160:A9807.

41. Mahmud E, Behnamfar O, Ang L, Patel MP, Poch D, Kim NH. Balloon pulmonary angioplasty for chronic thromboembolic pulmonary hypertension. Interv Cardiol Clin. 2018;7(1):103–17.

42. Danilov NM, Matchin YG, Chernyavsky AM, Edemsky AG, Grankin DS, Sagaydak OV, et al. Balloon pulmonary angioplasty for patients with inoperable chronic thromboembolic pulmonary hypertension. Ter Arkh. 2019;91(4):43–7.

43. Sepúlveda P, Ortega J, Armijo G, Torres J, Ramírez P, Backhouse C, et al. Balloon pulmonary angioplasty for the treatment of chronic thromboembolic pulmonary hypertension. Rev Med Chil. 2019;147(4):426–36.

44. Hoole SP, Coghlan JG, Cannon JE, Taboada D, Toshner M, Sheares K, et al. Balloon pulmonary angioplasty for inoperable chronic thromboembolic pulmonary hypertension: the UK experience. Open heart. 2020;7(1):e001144.

45. Karyofyllis P, Tsiapras D, Papadopoulou V, Diamantidis MD, Fotiou P, Demerouti E, et al. Balloon pulmonary angioplasty is a promising option in thalassemic patients with inoperable chronic

thromboembolic pulmonary hypertension. J Thromb Thrombolysis. 2018;46(4):516–20.

46. Tanabe N, Kawakami T, Satoh T, Matsubara H, Nakanishi N, Ogino H, et al. Balloon pulmonary angioplasty for chronic thromboembolic pulmonary hypertension: a systematic review. Respir Investig. 2018;56(4):332–41.

47. Zoppellaro G, Badawy MR, Squizzato A, Denas G, Tarantini G, Pengo V. Balloon pulmonary angioplasty in patients with chronic thromboembolic pulmonary hypertension - a systematic review and meta-analysis. Circulation. 2019;83(8):1660–7.

48. Khan MS, Amin E, Memon MM, Yamani N, Siddiqi TJ, Khan SU, et al. Meta-analysis of use of balloon pulmonary angioplasty in patients with inoperable chronic thromboembolic pulmonary hypertension. Int J Cardiol. 2019;2019:5.

49. Anand V, Frantz RP, DuBrock H, Kane GC, Krowka M, Yanagisawa R, et al. Balloon pulmonary angioplasty for chronic thromboembolic pulmonary hypertension: initial single-center experience. Mayo Clinic Proc Innov Qual Outcomes. 2019;3(3):311–8.

50. Jin Q, Luo Q, Yang T, Zeng Q, Yu X, Yan L, et al. Improved hemodynamics and cardiopulmonary function in patients with inoperable chronic thromboembolic pulmonary hypertension after balloon pulmonary angioplasty. Respir Res. 2019;20(1):250.

51. Akizuki M, Serizawa N, Ueno A, Adachi T, Hagiwara N. Effect of balloon pulmonary angioplasty on respiratory function in patients with chronic thromboembolic pulmonary hypertension. Chest. 2017;151(3):643–9.

52. Tsugu T, Murata M, Kawakami T, Minakata Y, Kanazawa H, Kataoka M, et al. Changes in right ventricular dysfunction after balloon pulmonary angioplasty in patients with chronic thromboembolic pulmonary hypertension. Am J Cardiol. 2016;118(7):1081–7.

53. Kanar BG, Mutlu B, Atas H, Akaslan D, Yıldızeli B. Improvements of right ventricular function and hemodynamics after balloon pulmonary angioplasty in patients with chronic thromboembolic pulmonary hypertension. Echocardiography. 2019;36(11):2050–6.

54. Yamasaki Y, Nagao M, Abe K, Hosokawa K, Kawanami S, Kamitani T, et al. Balloon pulmonary angioplasty improves interventricular dyssynchrony in patients with inoperable chronic thromboembolic pulmonary hypertension: a cardiac MR imaging study. Int J Cardiovasc Imaging. 2017;33(2):229–39.

55. Kriechbaum SD, Wiedenroth CB, Hesse ML, Ajnwojner R, Keller T, Sebastian Wolter J, et al. Development of renal function during staged balloon pulmonary angioplasty for inoperable chronic thromboembolic pulmonary hypertension. Scand J Clin Lab Invest. 2019;79(4):268–75.

56. Darocha S, Banaszkiewicz M, Pietrasik A, Siennicka A, Piorunek M, Grochowska E, et al. Changes in estimated glomerular filtration after balloon pulmonary angioplasty for chronic thromboembolic pulmonary hypertension. Cardiorenal Med. 2020;10(1):22–31.

57. Nakamura M, Sunagawa O, Tsuchiya H, Miyara T, Taba Y, Touma T, et al. Rescue balloon pulmonary angioplasty under veno-arterial extracorporeal membrane oxygenation in a patient with acute exacerbation of chronic thromboembolic pulmonary hypertension. Int Heart J. 2015;56(1):116–20.

58. Collaud S, Brenot P, Mercier O, Fadel E. Rescue balloon pulmonary angioplasty for early failure of pulmonary endarterectomy: the earlier the better? Int J Cardiol. 2016;222:39–40.

59. Wiedenroth CB, Liebetrau C, Breithecker A, Guth S, Lautze HJ, Ortmann E, et al. Combined pulmonary endarterectomy and balloon pulmonary angioplasty in patients with chronic thromboembolic pulmonary hypertension. J Heart Lung Transplant. 2016;35(5):591–6.

60. Godinas L, Bonne L, Budts W, Belge C, Leys M, Delcroix M, et al. Balloon pulmonary angioplasty for the treatment of nonoperable chronic thromboembolic pulmonary hypertension: single-center experience with low initial complication rate. J Vasc Interv Radiol. 2019;30(8):1265–72.

61. Araszkiewicz A, Darocha S, Pietrasik A, Pietura R, Jankiewicz S, Banaszkiewicz M, et al. Balloon pulmonary angioplasty for the treatment of residual or recurrent pulmonary hypertension after pulmonary endarterectomy. Int J Cardiol. 2019;278:232–7.

62. Yanaka K, Nakayama K, Shinke T, Shinkura Y, Taniguchi Y, Kinutani H, et al. Sequential hybrid therapy with pulmonary endarterectomy and additional balloon pulmonary angioplasty for chronic thromboembolic pulmonary hypertension. J Am Heart Assoc. 2018;7:13.

63. Shimura N, Kataoka M, Inami T, Yanagisawa R, Ishiguro H, Kawakami T, et al. Additional percutaneous transluminal pulmonary angioplasty for residual or recurrent pulmonary hypertension after pulmonary endarterectomy. Int J Cardiol. 2015;183:138–42.

64. Inami T, Kataoka M, Kikuchi H, Goda A, Satoh T. Balloon pulmonary angioplasty for symptomatic chronic thromboembolic disease without pulmonary hypertension at rest. Int J Cardiol. 2019;289:116–8.

65. Wiedenroth CB, Olsson KM, Guth S, Breithecker A, Haas M, Kamp JC, et al. Balloon pulmonary angioplasty for inoperable patients with chronic thromboembolic disease. Pulmonary Circul. 2018;8(1):2045893217753122.

66. Taboada D, Pepke-Zaba J, Jenkins DP, Berman M, Treacy CM, Cannon JE, et al. Outcome of pulmonary endarterectomy in symptomatic chronic thromboembolic disease. Eur Respir J. 2014;44(6):1635–45.

67. Ejiri K, Ogawa A, Fujii S, Ito H, Matsubara H. Vascular injury is a major cause of lung injury after balloon pulmonary angioplasty in patients with chronic thromboembolic pulmonary hypertension. Circ Cardiovasc Interv. 2018;11(12):e005884.

68. Ikeda N, Kubota S, Okazaki T, Iijima R, Hara H, Hiroi Y, et al. The predictors of complications in balloon pulmonary angioplasty for chronic thromboembolic

pulmonary hypertension. Catheter Cardiovasc Interv. 2019;2019:1.

69. Kimura M, Kohno T, Kawakami T, Kataoka M, Hiraide T, Moriyama H, et al. Shortening hospital stay is feasible and safe in patients with chronic thromboembolic pulmonary hypertension treated with balloon pulmonary angioplasty. Can J Cardiol. 2019;35(2):193–8.

70. Mahmud E, Madani MM, Kim NH, Poch D, Ang L, Behnamfar O, et al. Chronic thromboembolic pulmo-

nary hypertension: evolving therapeutic approaches for operable and inoperable disease. J Am Coll Cardiol. 2018;71(21):2468–86.

71. Takei M, Kawakami T, Kataoka M, Kuwahira I, Fukuda K. Residual high intrapulmonary shunt fraction limits exercise capacity in patients treated with balloon pulmonary angioplasty. Heart Vessels. 2019;34(5):868–74.

Lesion Classification in Chronic Thromboembolic Pulmonary Hypertension from an Interventional Perspective

7

Marcin Kurzyna, Szymon Darocha, Marta Banaszkiewicz-Cyganik, and Adam Torbicki

7.1 Introduction

Vascular lesions that cause increased pulmonary vascular resistance in CTEPH are themselves caused by organized thrombi persisting in the lungs after episodes of acute pulmonary embolism. While some such thrombi completely occlude one or more of the pulmonary arterial branches, in most cases some degree of recanalization is present. The recanalization process varies from patient to patient and from vessel to vessel in the same patient, as does the morphology of vascular lesions. Typically, the vascular lesion pattern in a patient undergoing BPA is a mixture of different lesion types, and CTEPH is always a multivessel disease from an interventional treatment standpoint. Thrombi, traveling to the lungs during acute embolism, are usually stuck at the vessels' bifurcations, so that vascular lesions in CTEPH in more than 80% involve bifurcations. There is an apparent predominance of the frequency of CTEPH-specific lesions in the right lung relative to the left lung and the

M. Kurzyna (✉) · S. Darocha
M. Banaszkiewicz-Cyganik · A. Torbicki
Department of Pulmonary Circulation, Thromboembolic Diseases and Cardiology, Centre for Postgraduate Medical Education in Warsaw, European Health Centre, Otwock, Poland
e-mail: marcin.kurzyna@ecz-otwock.pl; szymon. darocha@ecz-otwock.pl; marta.banaszkiewicz@ecz-otwock.pl; adam.torbicki@ecz-otwock.pl

lower lobes relative to the upper lobes. The formation of anastomoses between the bronchial arteries and peripheral branches of the pulmonary arteries helps to preserve the patency in their distal segments, which is essential for effective interventional treatment but may increase the risk of bleeding. Similar to coronary interventions, evaluation of vascular lesions in CTEPH according to a standardized classification may improve the accuracy of qualification for surgical and percutaneous treatment and the overall efficacy and safety of therapy [1].

7.2 Surgical Classification of Vascular Lesions in CTEPH

The surgical classification of vascular lesions found in CTEPH mainly focuses on the proximal part of the thrombus relevant to the initiation of the endarterectomy plane during the surgical procedure. According to the classification proposed by a San Diego group, the vascular lesions are divided into four levels according to the location of the proximal part of the thrombus, separately for each lung [2]. Level I represents thrombi beginning at the level of the main pulmonary arteries, level II represents thrombi located in the lobar arteries, and levels III and IV represent thrombi located in the segmental and subsegmental arteries, respectively. According to their anatomic disease operability, levels I and II are assumed to be unequivocally operable lesions. In contrast, level IV includes lesions located too distally for surgical access. Level III disease remains an overlap zone where good results can be achieved with both surgical and interventional treatment [3, 4].

The choice of appropriate treatment for disease defined as level III depends largely on the local surgical and interventional teams' experience. The decision should be worked out during a CTEPH team meeting [5]. The usefulness of the described classification for interventional treatment planning is limited because it focuses on determining the thrombus's proximal location, which may not reflect the most significant part of the vascular resistance, perhaps due to numerous other vascular lesions located more distally. The above classification does not consider the relationship between the severity of the thrombotic load and pulmonary vascular resistance, which is an important element of preoperative assessment and must be subjectively evaluated.

7.3 Morphological Classification of Vascular Lesions in CTEPH: Tomographic Imaging Techniques in the Cathlab

Pulmonary angiography is still considered the gold standard for imaging in CTEPH diagnosis. In clinical practice, preoperative imaging of pulmonary artery lesions is usually performed using digital subtraction angiography (DSA) and computed tomography pulmonary angiography. However, such procedures might not be precise enough to evaluate lesions within the subsegmental branches. Cone beam computed tomography (CBCT), being a three-dimensional, high-spatial-resolution imaging technique, yields purer images of lesions in subsegmental arteries than conventional methods. Hinrichs et al. compared CBCT with DSA and found at CBCT derived images of the central and peripheral pulmonary arteries, findings missed on DSA. The authors considered a more comprehensive evaluation of pulmonary arteries concerning bands, webs, and intraluminal stenoses using CBCT. Therefore,

CBCT images might influence patient selection for interventional treatment [6]. Fukuda et al. evaluated the feasibility of CBCT during pulmonary angiography in terms of preoperative simulation of BPA. They classified CTEPH lesions assessed by CBCT into five subtypes for planning the BPA procedure, viz.: type 1a—webs; type 1b—web with severe narrowing of the subsegmental artery; type 2—webs and slits; type 3—slits; and type 4—pouch defect with incomplete obstruction of subsegmental branches or complete occlusion of subsegmental branches. CBCT findings were consistent with those obtained in wedged or selective angiography in 92.6% within subsegmental branches, and consistent with findings obtained in conventional angiography only in 27.6%. In detail, 85% of branches containing type 1, 2, or 3 lesions were appropriately assessed for treatment using CBCT before BPA, while only 5% were correctly assessed using conventional angiography only. In terms of BPA safety, type 1a and type 2 lesions were indicated as promising candidates for the first procedure of BPA. In contrast, type 1b and type IV lesions should be selected for further stages of treatment after achieving a decrease in mean pulmonary artery pressure (Fig. 7.1) [7].

In a subsequent study, Ogo et al. assessed 385 sessions of BPA guided by CBCT or electrocardiogram-gated area detector CT (ADCT) in terms of efficacy and complications. They concluded that pre-BPA assessment of webs and slits as target lesions by CBCT or ADCT, with the avoidance of angioplasty for complete obstructive lesions, might be important as an effective and safe interventional treatment strategy [8]. However, there is still a need for novel visualization techniques that would accurately reflect the complex anatomy of the pulmonary artery with regard to the three-dimensional relationship between structures. Three-dimensional (3D) printing and augmented reality (AR) are considered emerging tools, useful in navigation planning and guiding of transcatheter pulmonary interventions, as reported by Witkowski et al. [9]. The authors presented effective use of pulmonary vascular tree holograms prepared with Microsoft HoloLens AR headsets.

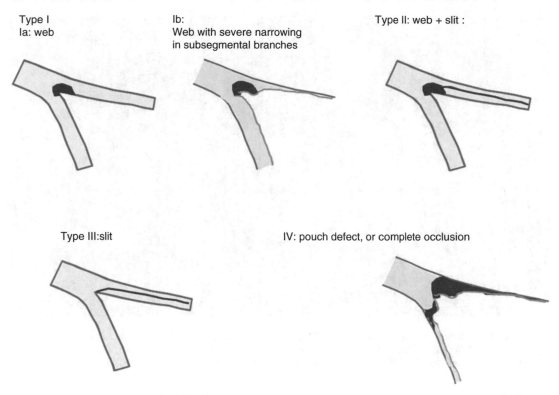

Type I
Ia: web

Ib:
Web with severe narrowing
in subsegmental branches

Type II: web + slit :

Type III:slit

IV: pouch defect, or complete occlusion

Fig. 7.1 Schematic representation of organized thrombi assessed with cone beam computed tomography. Type 1a—webs; type 1b—web with severe narrowing of subsegmental artery; type 2—web and slits; type 3—slits; and type 4—pouch defect with incomplete obstruction of subsegmental branches or complete occlusion. From Fukuda et al., Jpn. J. Radiol, 2016 with permission [7]

Additionally, 3D printed life-sized models of the same structures were prepared for preoperative planning. Augmented reality in BPA technique improvement might be related to better target lesion selections, improved balloon catheter sizing, decreased volume of contrast medium, and more extensive revascularization (Fig. 7.2).

7.4 Morphological Classification of Vascular Lesions in CTEPH: Intravascular Imaging

Morphological assessment of vascular lesions in CTEPH is possible by direct evaluation with angioscopy or by visualization with intravascular imaging techniques. According to Inohara et al., optical coherence tomography (OCT) provides images that show the morphology of vascular lesions better than intravascular ultrasound (IVUS) [10]. The authors proposed a classification based on the morphology of the vascular lesions assessed by OCT. Vascular lesions were classified as a mono-hole, septum, multi-hole with thin walls, and multi-hole with thick walls (Fig. 7.3). The authors did not find a clear correlation between the morphology of lesions assessed by OCT and angiographic presentation. For example, the multi-hole lesions were present in all angiographic patterns. The therapeutic effect of BPA was most pronounced in multi-hole and septum lesions and least pronounced in mono-hole lesions.

A similar classification based on OCT was presented by Ishiguro et al. [11], who defined four types of vascular lesions according to the number of channels and volume of intravascular septa. Lesions may be a ringlike obstruction or

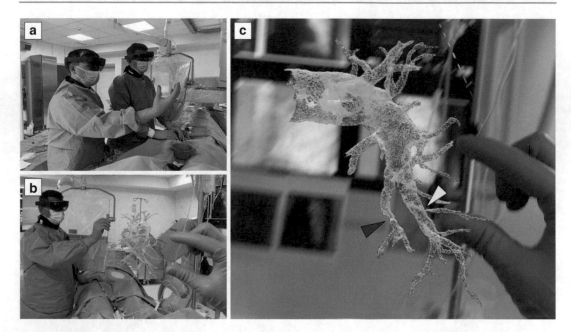

Fig. 7.2 BPA supported by Augmented Reality. Operators using Microsoft HoloLens® AR headsets with CarnaLife Holo® software (**a**: side view). A presentation of left pulmonary artery hologram (**b**: operator's view). Panel **c**: Selection of targeted web lesion (red arrow) and narrowed branch in ostium (yellow arrow)

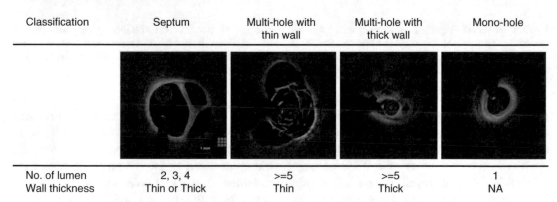

Classification	Septum	Multi-hole with thin wall	Multi-hole with thick wall	Mono-hole
No. of lumen	2, 3, 4	>=5	>=5	1
Wall thickness	Thin or Thick	Thin	Thick	NA

Fig. 7.3 Demonstration of the OCT-based classification of CTEPH: [1] septum, [2] multi-hole with thin wall, [3] multi-hole with thick wall, [4] mono-hole. "Septum" indicated that a partition separated the lumen into less than four components. "Multi-hole with thin wall" referred to the mesh-like flaps in the lumen, which separated the lumen into more than five components, and the flaps were thin. "Multi-hole with thick wall" demonstrated the occu-pied thrombus in the lumen with several channels. As with "multi-hole with thin wall," this type had more than five components in the lumen, but the partition walls were thicker than those of the "multi-hole with thin wall" type. "Mono-hole" denoted the occupied thrombus in the lumen with a single small channel. From Inohara et al. Int J Cardiol 2015 with permission [10]

had a honeycomb-like structure. In more com-plex lesions, the OCT revealed a lotus rootlike structure, which was difficult to identify by angiography but relatively easy to tear down by balloon dilation. In the last type, the OCT dem-onstrated a lotus rootlike structure within the ves-sel, with an organized thrombus adhering to the vessel wall.

Due to the relatively rare use of OCT during BPA procedures, morphological classifications based on this technique have not been widely adopted in clinical practice. Nevertheless, the

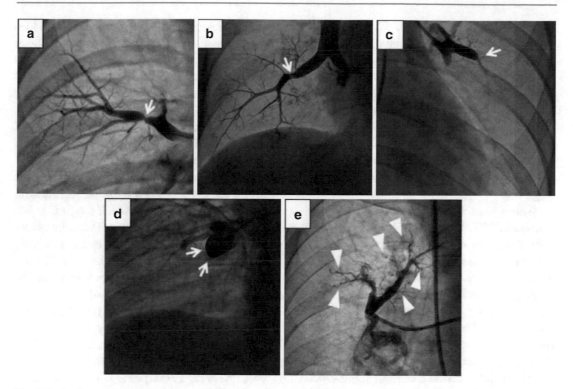

Fig. 7.4 Angiographic classification of lesion morphology based on the lesion opacity and the blood flow distal to the lesion. (**a**) Ringlike stenosis lesion. (**b**) Web lesion. (**c**) Subtotal lesion. (**d**) Total occlusion lesion. (**e**) Tortuous lesion. From Kawakami et al, Circ Cardiovasc Interv, 2016 with permission [13]

knowledge of vascular lesion morphology obtained from OCT improves the understanding of CTEPH and the therapeutic effect of BPA [12].

7.5 Lesion Quantification Based on Selective Pulmonary Angiography

Kawakami et al. [13] evaluated 1936 vascular lesions treated with BPA during 500 procedures performed in 97 patients with CTEPH. They proposed a classification that divided vascular lesions in CTEPH into five categories: ringlike stenosis (type A), web lesion (type B), subtotal occlusion (type C), total occlusion (type D), and tortuous lesion (type E). This classification is currently the basis for evaluating vascular lesions eligible for BPA and groups vascular lesions according to their appearance on angiography to determine percutaneous treatment availability,

intervention tactics, risk of complications, and expected therapeutic outcomes (Fig. 7.4).

Ringlike stenosis (type A) accounts for approximately 13% of lesions treated with BPA. Ringlike stenoses are located mostly at the orifice of side branches from the main vascular trunks, so it is often impossible to measure the vessel diameter proximally to the lesion. If it can be done, it does not differ from the reference diameter beyond the stenosis. The stenosis itself is relatively short, and it can be challenging to assess its significance by angiography. Also, the use of intravascular imaging techniques like IVUS or OCT may not be conclusive about the lesion's hemodynamic significance. In the case of ringlike lesions, functional assessment by measuring the pressure gradient across the lesion may be helpful. Ringlike lesions can be easily crossed with a vascular guide, and the risk of complications when passing through the lesion is negligible. The balloon catheter size used for angioplasty should be guided by the diameter of the distal reference segment. Sizing of the balloon catheter 1:1 with the distal reference usually provides a safe and effective BPA.

Web lesions (type B) are the most common type of vascular lesions that undergo BPA and occur in over 60% of all treated lesions. They have highly variable morphology and may present as long structures extending along the vessel, short segments with discrete translucency, or abrupt narrowing of the vessel's distal portion (Fig. 7.5).

Web lesions are the longest type of vascular lesions in CTEPH and usually occur in smaller caliber vessels than ringlike lesions. Assessing the hemodynamic significance of web lesions is usually not very difficult, although it can be challenging in short lesions which are not clearly visible on angiography. An essential part of assessing a web-like lesion's significance is the evaluation of flow in the vessel's distal part. Also, low parenchymal perfusion and poor venous return provide additional information about the significance of the stenosis. Standard types of vascular guidewires are suitable for crossing a type B lesion, and the success rate is over 95%. The most common complication is wire injury, so care must be taken to place the guidewire deep in the vessel's distal portion to ensure that it is in the main channel of the treated vessel. Difficulties with guidewire passage are most commonly associated with entering one of the "blind" channels of web lesion or small side branch penetration. When choosing the diameter of a balloon catheter, the presence of connective tissue forming an intra-

vascular mesh should be kept in mind. In lesions with a massive tissue component, the catheter diameter reduction in relation to the reference segment should be more considerable. Tapered balloon catheters may be applicable in dilating long web lesions.

Subtotal occlusions (type C) take the form of significant and abrupt stenosis with preserved trace flow in the distal portion of the vessel and account for approximately 20% of lesions selected for BPA. The distal, subpleural segment is usually not visible (Fig. 7.6). If a type C lesion cannot be crossed with a standard vascular guidewire, a hydrophilic coated guidewire with a tip load between 1.0 and 1.5 g can be used. The use of CTO guidewires with high tip load should be reserved for exceptional cases [14].

During treatment of complex type C lesions, a high incidence of wire injury complications exceeding 10% should be expected. If a distal segment of the vessel is not visible, a guide extension catheter or IVUS probe can be used additionally. The use of a guide extension catheter enables the administration of contrast into the distal part of the vessel to ensure the set's position. Similarly, the use of IVUS confirms the position inside the vessel's lumen. Dilation of subtotal occlusion lesions should start with small balloon catheter diameters, i.e., 2.0–2.5 mm. Optimization should be deferred until the next procedural session because, after initial dilatation of the treated lesion, the vessel's distal portion usually increases in diameter once blood flow is restored.

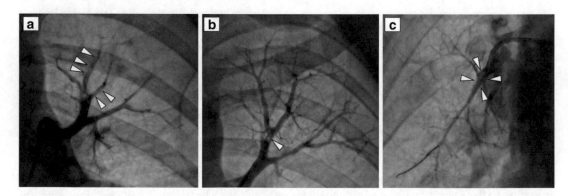

Fig. 7.5 Examples of web lesion: angiographic presentation as longitudinal defect (**a**), complex mesh (**b**), or abrupt narrowing (**c**) within the vessel

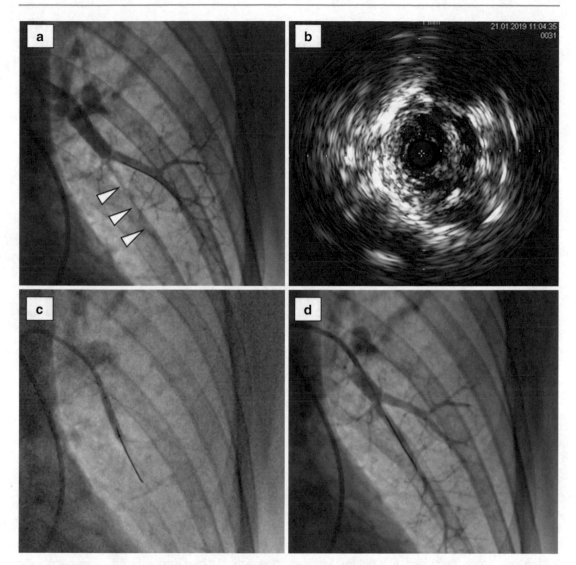

Fig. 7.6 Balloon pulmonary angioplasty of subtotal occlusion (type C lesion) in one of the lingular branches of the left lung. Selective angiography presents subtotal occlusion (arrows) of the subsegmental branch of the left pulmonary artery (**a**). Organized web lesion presented on IVUS examination (**b**). Inflation of balloon catheter in the ostium (**c**). The final effect of BPA presented on angiography (**d**)

Total occlusions (type D), otherwise known as pouch lesions, account for less than 5% of lesions and occur most commonly at the level of the segmental arteries. The low incidence of type D lesions in patients undergoing BPA procedures results from the fact that they are usually treated with surgery. They should be expected to occur in patients rejected from pulmonary endarterectomy because of comorbidities or those who do not consent to surgery. They are characterized by complete occlusion with no evidence of distal flow. Occasionally, the vessel's distal part is filled from the collateral circulation from adjacent branches of the pulmonary artery. The antegrade revascularization of pouch-type lesions requires considerable experience. It should be performed in the final stages of the treatment process when more easily accessible vascular lesions have all been treated as well as when pulmonary artery pressure has been reduced as much as possible. The guiding catheter's shape should be selected to allow its axial alignment with the visible vessel stump or its distal portion's anticipated course. Occasionally, a trace of distal flow may be visualized after contrast injection in the lesion's immediate vicinity. By operating with a guiding catheter near the lesion, a controlled attempt can be made to detach the thrombus from the vessel wall gently and thus visualize the distal portion of the vessel [15]. A guidewire dedicated to treating CTO lesions with high tip load or a soft hydrophilic guidewire can be used to force through the pouch lesion, counting on its penetration of the preserved flow channel. Single cases of the retrograde approach of type D lesions in the presence of extensive collaterals have been described [16, 17]. After unblocking, the possibility of elastic recoil must be anticipated due to the large bulk of thrombi causing type D lesion, which may require the implantation of a vascular stent in selected cases [18]. The reported low complication rates associated with the treatment of type D lesions are mainly due to the inability to overcome the lesion with the guidewire.

Tortuous lesions (type E) are located in the terminal branches of subsegmental arteries with a diameter of 2–3 mm. They are characterized by a tortuous course near the capillary bed. The risk of wire injury during treatment of type E lesions is most significant at over 40%. Soft, hydrophobic guidewires and small-diameter balloon catheters are recommended. Manipulation of the instrumentation should be meticulous, taking into account respiratory movements and heartbeat, which may move the guidewire's tip. For a therapeutic effect, many dilatations should be performed due to the small-vessel calibers. Given that patients with predominantly tortuous lesions initially have high pressure and pulmonary resistance values, the final effect is usually low.

A separate category of vascular lesions that undergo BPA is lesions in vessels after earlier surgical pulmonary endarterectomy (PEA). These lesions are usually located at the level of the subsegmental arteries and begin abruptly at the sites where the intima with or without an adjacent organized thrombus is detached. Movable flaps can be seen in the vessel lumen at these sites. Typically, lesions seen in patients after PEA can be of type B, C, and D. Residual

CTEPH after PEA can be effectively treated with BPA [19–21]. Nevertheless, more caution should be paid with guiding catheter manipulation because proximal to post-PEA lesion vessels lack an intimal and medial membrane and this favors the formation of dilatation and aneurysms (Fig. 7.7).

7.6 Post-BPA Evolution of Vascular Lesions

The mechanism of how permanent dilatation of the pulmonary arterial lumen occurs after BPA is not fully elucidated, given that the tissue forming intravascular obstructions is not evacuated from the vessel as is the case in PEA. Shimokawahara et al. evaluated with IVUS 326 vascular lesions treated during 220 BPA procedures. The lesions were of the ringlike (type A), web (type B), and subtotal occlusion (type C) types. On baseline IVUS assessment, the area occupied by thrombotic tissue differed across all lesion types—it was smallest in type A lesions (65.5%), more extensive in type B lesions (72.5%), and largest in type C lesions (82.2%). After BPA, in all lesion types, an enlargement of the flow lumen associated with a widening of the vessel's outer diameter was recorded, which was evident regardless of the lesion type. There was a positive correlation between the increase in the arterial lumen and the vessel's outer diameter. In contrast, compression of the elastic-fibrotic component was seen only in type B and type C lesions but was absent in type A lesions [22]. Magoń et al., in a study evaluating the effect of 98 dilation of ringlike (type A) and web lesions (type B) using IVUS and virtual histology, demonstrated that the vessel stretch mechanism was more pronounced in larger vessels, whereas compression of fibrous thrombus-forming connective tissue predominated in smaller vessels. The authors explained this difference by the decreasing content of elastic fibers with reduction in vessel diameter [23].

An additional mechanism accompanying dilation of vascular lesions during BPA is local dissection due to detachment of fibrotic elements

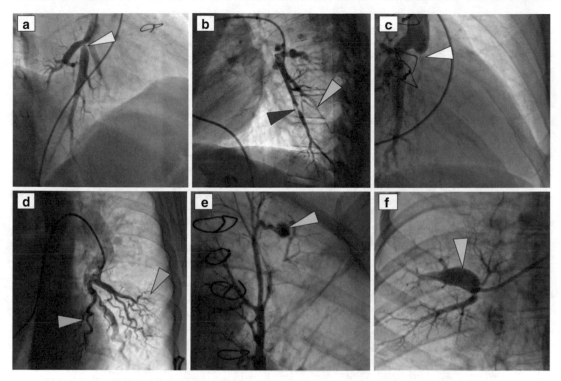

Fig. 7.7 Types of thromboembolic lesions and vascular changes found in selected patients with persistent CTEPH after PEA. Panel **a**: ringlike stenosis. Panel **b**: webs and bands (red arrow) and subtotal occlusion (orange arrow). Panel **c**: total occlusion (pouch lesion). Panel **d**: pulmonary microangiopathy, tortuous and "corkscrewed" ves- sels (blue arrows). Panel **e**: pulmonary artery anastomoses connected to collateral circulation (green arrow). Panel **f**: post-stenotic aneurysm (ectasia) of pulmonary artery (gray arrow). From Araszkiewicz et al. Int. J. Cardiol, 2019 with permission [19]

from the vessel wall. It can be speculated that the greatest risk of unfavorable dilation may be present in type B and C lesions, where the ratio of fibrotic material to total vessel cross-sectional area is highest [24]. The presence of small dissections within the vessel wall may promote discrete bleeding that is not apparent during the procedure but manifests several hours later as reperfusion lung injury. The dissections described above have a natural tendency to self-heal; nevertheless, repeated inflation with catheters of increased diameter at the same site should be avoided. Some authors recommend reducing the balloon catheter diameter to 80% of the vessel diameter in web lesions and to 60% in type C lesions when the mean pulmonary artery pressure is below 35 mmHg. If the mean pulmonary artery pressure exceeds 35 mmHg, the suggested balloon catheter diameter should be 60% and 50% of the vessel lumen in type B and C lesions, respectively [25].

7.7   Summary

Several classifications of vascular lesions in CTEPH utilize different imaging techniques, but the assessment based on selective pulmonary angiography seems to be the most useful and practical. The degree of vessel stenosis in CTEPH is not a sufficient criterion for assessing the significance of vascular lesions because of their morphological diversity. The use of systematic classification with a documented relationship with efficacy and safety of BPA facilitates treatment selection by the CTEPH team. The classification of vascular lesions successfully allows the determination of the procedure's difficulty and the risk of complications. At the BPA planning stage, classification facilitates the selection of vessels which should be treated first. If high-risk lesions are present, vascular lesion classification can hasten treatment decisions at a more experienced center.

References

1. Sianos G, Morel MA, Kappetein AP, Morice MC, Colombo A, Dawkins K, et al. The SYNTAX score: an angiographic tool grading the complexity of coronary artery disease. EuroIntervention. 2005;1(2):219–27.
2. Madani MM. Surgical treatment of chronic thromboembolic pulmonary hypertension: pulmonary Thromboendarterectomy. Methodist Debakey Cardiovasc J. 2016;12(4):213–8.
3. Darocha S, Araszkiewicz A, Kurzyna M, Banaszkiewicz M, Jankiewicz S, Dobosiewicz A, et al. Balloon pulmonary angioplasty in technically operable and technically inoperable chronic thromboembolic pulmonary hypertension. J Clin Med. 2021;10:1038.
4. Madani M, Ogo T, Simonneau G. The changing landscape of chronic thromboembolic pulmonary hypertension management. Eur Respir Rev. 2017;26:146.
5. Siennicka A, Darocha S, Banaszkiewicz M, Kedzierski P, Dobosiewicz A, Blaszczak P, et al. Treatment of chronic thromboembolic pulmonary hypertension in a multidisciplinary team. Ther Adv Respir Dis. 2019;13:1753466619891529.
6. Hinrichs JB, Marquardt S, von Falck C, Hoeper MM, Olsson KM, Wacker FK, et al. Comparison of C-arm computed tomography and digital subtraction angiography in patients with chronic thromboembolic pulmonary hypertension. Cardiovasc Intervent Radiol. 2016;39(1):53–63.
7. Fukuda T, Ogo T, Nakanishi N, Ueda J, Sanda Y, Morita Y, et al. Evaluation of organized thrombus in distal pulmonary arteries in patients with chronic thromboembolic pulmonary hypertension using cone-beam computed tomography. Jpn J Radiol. 2016;34(6):423–31.
8. Ogo T, Fukuda T, Tsuji A, Fukui S, Ueda J, Sanda Y, et al. Efficacy and safety of balloon pulmonary angioplasty for chronic thromboembolic pulmonary hypertension guided by cone-beam computed tomography and electrocardiogram-gated area detector computed tomography. Eur J Radiol. 2017;89:270–6.
9. Witowski J, Darocha S, Kownacki Ł, Pietrasik A, Pietura R, Banaszkiewicz M, et al. Augmented reality and three-dimensional printing in percutaneous interventions on pulmonary arteries. Quant Imaging Med Surg. 2018;9(1):23–9.
10. Inohara T, Kawakami T, Kataoka M, Yamamoto M, Kimura M, Kanazawa H, et al. Lesion morphological classification by OCT to predict therapeutic efficacy after balloon pulmonary angioplasty in CTEPH. Int J Cardiol. 2015;197:23–5.
11. Ishiguro H, Kataoka M, Inami T, Shimura N, Yanagisawa R, Kawakami T, et al. Diversity of lesion morphology in CTEPH analyzed by OCT, pressure wire, and angiography. JACC Cardiovasc Imaging. 2016;9(3):324–5.
12. Araszkiewicz A, Jankiewicz S, Lanocha M, Janus M, Mularek-Kubzdela T, Lesiak M. Optical coherence tomography improves the results of balloon pulmonary angioplasty in inoperable chronic thrombo-embolic pulmonary hypertension. Postepy Kardiol Interwencyjnej. 2017;13(2):180–1.
13. Kawakami T, Ogawa A, Miyaji K, Mizoguchi H, Shimokawahara H, Naito T, et al. Novel angiographic classification of each vascular lesion in chronic thromboembolic pulmonary hypertension based on selective angiogram and results of balloon pulmonary angioplasty. Circ Cardiovasc Interv. 2016;9:10.
14. Kurzyna M, Darocha S, Pietura R, Pietrasik A, Norwa J, Manczak R, et al. Changing the strategy of balloon pulmonary angioplasty resulted in a reduced complication rate in patients with chronic thromboembolic pulmonary hypertension. A single-centre European experience. Kardiol Pol. 2017;75(7):645–54.
15. Minatsuki S, Hatano M, Maki H, Ando J, Komuro I. The structure of a chronic total occlusion and its safe treatment in a patient with chronic thromboembolic pulmonary hypertension. Int Heart J. 2017;58(5):824–7.
16. Allen Ligon R, Petit CJ. Working backward: retrograde balloon angioplasty of atretic arteries in chronic thromboembolic pulmonary hypertension. Catheter Cardiovasc Interv. 2019;93(6):1076–9.
17. Kawakami T, Kataoka M, Arai T, Yanagisawa R, Maekawa Y, Fukuda K. Retrograde approach in balloon pulmonary angioplasty: useful novel strategy for chronic Total occlusion lesions in pulmonary arteries. JACC Cardiovasc Interv. 2016;9(2):e19–20.
18. Darocha S, Pietura R, Banaszkiewicz M, Pietrasik A, Kownacki L, Torbicki A, et al. Balloon pulmonary angioplasty with stent implantation as a treatment of proximal chronic thromboembolic pulmonary hypertension. Diagnostics. 2020;10:6.
19. Araszkiewicz A, Darocha S, Pietrasik A, Pietura R, Jankiewicz S, Banaszkiewicz M, et al. Balloon pulmonary angioplasty for the treatment of residual or recurrent pulmonary hypertension after pulmonary endarterectomy. Int J Cardiol. 2019;278:232–7.
20. Kopec G, Stepniewski J, Waligora M, Kurzyna M, Biederman A, Podolec P. Staged treatment of central and peripheral lesions in chronic thromboembolic pulmonary hypertension. Pol Arch Med Wewn. 2016;126(1–2):97–9.
21. Shimura N, Kataoka M, Inami T, Yanagisawa R, Ishiguro H, Kawakami T, et al. Additional percutaneous transluminal pulmonary angioplasty for residual or recurrent pulmonary hypertension after pulmonary endarterectomy. Int J Cardiol. 2015;183:138–42.
22. Shimokawahara H, Ogawa A, Mizoguchi H, Yagi H, Ikemiyagi H, Matsubara H. Vessel stretching is a cause of lumen enlargement immediately after balloon pulmonary angioplasty: intravascular ultrasound analysis in patients with chronic thromboembolic pulmonary hypertension. Circ Cardiovasc Interv. 2018;11(4):e006010.
23. Magon W, Stepniewski J, Waligora M, Jonas K, Przybylski R, Sikorska M, et al. Virtual histology to evaluate mechanisms of pulmonary artery lumen

enlargement in response to balloon pulmonary angioplasty in chronic thromboembolic pulmonary hypertension. J Clin Med. 2020;9:6.

24. Kitani M, Ogawa A, Sarashina T, Yamadori I, Matsubara H. Histological changes of pulmonary arteries treated by balloon pulmonary angioplasty in a patient with chronic thromboembolic pulmonary hypertension. Circ Cardiovasc Interv. 2014;7(6):857–9.

25. Roik M, Wretowski D, Labyk A, Kostrubiec M, Irzyk K, Dzikowska-Diduch O, et al. Refined balloon pulmonary angioplasty driven by combined assessment of intra-arterial anatomy and physiology—multimodal approach to treated lesions in patients with non-operable distal chronic thromboembolic pulmonary hypertension—Technique, safety and efficacy of 50 consecutive angioplasties. Int J Cardiol. 2016;203:228–35.

Advanced Noninvasive Imaging to Guide Balloon Pulmonary Angioplasty

Shigefumi Fukui, Koichiro Sugimura, Hideki Ota,
Satoshi Higuchi, Nobuhiro Yaoita, Tatsuo Aoki,
Yoshiaki Morita, Takeshi Ogo, Tetsuya Fukuda,
Kei Takase, Hiroaki Shimokawa,
and Satoshi Yasuda

S. Fukui (✉)
Department of Cardiovascular Medicine, Tohoku
University Graduate School of Medicine,
Sendai, Japan

Department of Cardiovascular Medicine, National
Cerebral and Cardiovascular Centre, Suita, Japan

Department of Cardiovascular Medicine, Tohoku
Medical and Pharmaceutical University,
Sendai, Japan
e-mail: sig-fuk@swan.ocn.ne.jp

K. Sugimura
Department of Cardiovascular Medicine, Tohoku
University Graduate School of Medicine,
Sendai, Japan

Department of Cardiology, International University
of Health and Welfare, Narita, Japan

H. Ota · K. Takase
Department of Diagnostic Radiology, Tohoku
University Graduate School of Medicine,
Sendai, Japan

S. Higuchi · Y. Morita
Department of Diagnostic Radiology, Tohoku
University Graduate School of Medicine,
Sendai, Japan

Department of Radiology, National Cerebral and
Cardiovascular Centre, Suita, Japan

N. Yaoita
Department of Cardiovascular Medicine, Tohoku
University Graduate School of Medicine,
Sendai, Japan

T. Aoki
Department of Cardiovascular Medicine, Tohoku
University Graduate School of Medicine,
Sendai, Japan

Department of Cardiovascular Medicine, National
Cerebral and Cardiovascular Centre, Suita, Japan

T. Ogo
Department of Cardiovascular Medicine, National
Cerebral and Cardiovascular Centre, Suita, Japan

T. Fukuda
Department of Radiology, National Cerebral and
Cardiovascular Centre, Suita, Japan

H. Shimokawa
Department of Cardiovascular Medicine, Tohoku
University Graduate School of Medicine,
Sendai, Japan

International University of Health and Welfare,
Narita, Japan

S. Yasuda
Department of Cardiovascular Medicine, Tohoku
University Graduate School of Medicine,
Sendai, Japan

Department of Cardiovascular Medicine, National
Cerebral and Cardiovascular Centre,
Suita, Japan

© Springer Nature Switzerland AG 2022
F. Saia et al. (eds.), *Balloon pulmonary angioplasty in patients with CTEPH*,
https://doi.org/10.1007/978-3-030-95997-5_8

8.1   Introduction

Balloon pulmonary angioplasty (BPA) was considered to be a highly invasive therapy around 2001, when Feinstein et al. reported that 1 of 18 patients who underwent BPA died from reperfusion pulmonary edema [1]. This result indicates a mortality rate of 5.6%, which was considered to be unacceptable compared to that of pulmonary endarterectomy (PEA) [1]. Actually, the pulmonary artery has many branches, and their relationship with each other is three-dimensionally complex and has many variations individually. It is difficult to sufficiently select and visualize the targeted vessels during BPA via selective angiography alone, which takes a long time and large amount of contrast agent to perform. Sometimes, we experience a misunderstanding of the position of a tip of a guide wire because of three-dimensionally overlapping vessels, especially when performing a BPA procedure with a single-plane setting, which may lead to a complication. In 2012, Mizoguchi and Matsubara et al., National Hospital Organization Okayama Medical Centre, demonstrated a refined, low-mortality BPA procedure that improved the clinical status and hemodynamics of patients with inoperable chronic thromboembolic pulmonary hypertension (CTEPH), using intravascular ultrasound (IVUS) [2]. Thereafter, several investigators have reported the efficacy of invasive (intravascular) and noninvasive imaging in order to improve BPA results, to reduce complications, and to evaluate the efficacy of BPA, such as a pressure wire; optical coherence tomography; computed tomography (CT) of three-dimensional (3D), 4D, cone-beam, C-arm, and electrocardiogram (ECG)-gated area detector; and dual-energy and cardiovascular magnetic resonance (CMR) of cine, 4D flow, and right atrial (RA) function [3–17]. From the view to technically guide BPA, it is important for BPA operators to have enough information in preparation from noninvasive imaging before starting a BPA procedure, which helps us to select targeted vessels or lesions, appropriate guide wire or guiding catheter, and the most suitable projection angle to distinguish targeted vessels from the three-dimensionally overlapping vessels, without loss of contrast agent and procedure time.

In this chapter, first, we would like to document previously published noninvasive imaging technique and then the current practice before and during a BPA procedure in our CTEPH team, by focusing on the two points of how to use noninvasive imaging to improve BPA technique, and how to evaluate BPA efficacy, using CT and CMR.

8.2   Previously Published Noninvasive Imaging Technique to Guide BPA

There have been a lot of publications related to noninvasive imaging technique to guide BPA as follows in chronological order. In 2014, Sugiyama, a member of our CTEPH team, and colleagues reported the usefulness of cone-beam CT (CBCT) performed during diagnostic pulmonary angiography for the evaluation of organized thrombi at segmental or subsegmental arteries before BPA in patients with CTEPH, although CBCT does not fully meet "noninvasiveness" from the viewpoint of the use of a catheter (Fig. 8.1) [7]. They compared conventional contrast-enhanced CT pulmonary angiography (CTPA) with 3D and a multiplanar reformation (MPR) image of CBCT in 13 patients with CTEPH, by adding reconstruction process of CBCT performed during pulmonary digital subtraction angiography (DSA), with the use of a 5 Fr. angled pigtail catheter. In their report, organized thrombi at subsegmental pulmonary arteries were more precisely evaluated by CBCT than CTPA, whereas those at segmental arteries are not so different between the two methods. In 2016, Fukuda, one of the leading members of our CTEPH team, and colleagues demonstrated in 32 patients with CTEPH the classification of typical CTEPH lesions consisting of five subtypes and also that 92.6% of the CTEPH lesions diagnosed by CBCT were highly consistent with the findings of selective angiography during BPA (Fig. 8.2) [8]. Thus, CBCT was found to be superior to conventional pulmonary DSA to identify

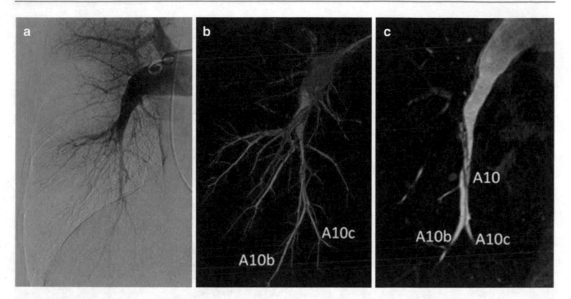

Fig. 8.1 Comparison of cone-beam computed tomography (CBCT) with pulmonary digital subtraction angiography (DSA) for the evaluation of organized thrombi. Representative image of DSA (**a**), a three dimension (**b**), and a multiplanar reformation (**c**) of CBCT for the right pulmonary artery in a 70-year-old woman with chronic thromboembolic pulmonary hypertension. This data is quoted from the reference No. 7

the lesion in the distal portion of the pulmonary arteries. Hinrichs et al. demonstrated in 52 patients with CTEPH comparison of ECG-gated DSA and contrast-enhanced C-arm computed tomography (CACT) that was obtained using a 5-F pigtail catheter by similar methods as CBCT [9]. They concluded that CACT of the pulmonary arteries is feasible and provides additional information by revealing abnormalities and findings missed on DSA alone. In 2017, Ogo, one of the leading members of our CTEPH team, and colleagues reported on 80 consecutive patients with inoperable CTEPH who received BPA guided by CBCT or ECG-gated area detector CT (ADCT) for target lesion assessment [11]. They concluded that ADCT image clearly showed the distal pulmonary artery and web formation, which are not well visible even in pulmonary DSA or selective angiography during BPA (Fig. 8.3). This seems to be a surprising finding, because we can obtain information about the form of webs, vessel diameter, and vessel running direction at more distal portion in the pulmonary arteries than levels visible in selective angiography, before starting a BPA procedure. This imaging from ADCT can help us to steer wire in order to pass through the tight webs, including a subtotal lesion and a

chronic total occlusion (CTO). In 2019, Maschke et al. assessed in 67 patients the frequency and severity of complications of BPA using CACT guidance, which was obtained during BPA sessions using catheter by similar methods as CBCT [18]. Briefly, after bone segmentation and subtraction, the CACT images were visualized as a 3D vascular tree by a volume rendering technique (VRT). In their report, 237 interventions were conducted without any complications (89.1%), with no fatal or life-threatening peri- or postinterventional complications or mortality. In 2020, Lin et al. reported the usefulness of DynaCT angiographic reconstruction guidance during BPA in their 23 patients with CTEPH [5]. More targeted vessels were treated in a single BPA procedure using the DynaCT angiographic reconstruction technique (3D group), compared to the DSA two-dimensional angiography (2D group), which was achieved in a shorter operation time. The use of the DynaCT angiographic reconstruction technique to guide BPA was also associated with a lower dose of contrast agent and less radiation exposure. In 2020, Tamura and Kawakami et al. reported the usefulness of time-resolved 4D CT angiography (4D CTA) to evaluate the bronchial artery-to-left inferior pul-

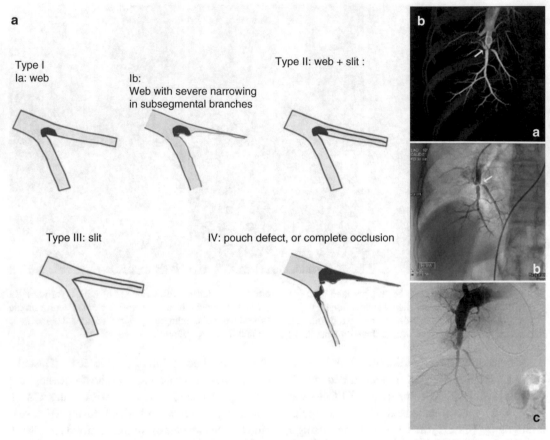

Fig. 8.2 Classification of typical chronic thromboembolic pulmonary hypertension (CTEPH) lesions consisting of five subtypes and consistency of cone-beam computed tomography (CBCT) with selective angiography during balloon pulmonary angioplasty (BPA). The classification of typical CTEPH lesions from type I to IV

(**a**). (**b**) Representative image of CBCT (**a**), selective angiography during BPA (**b**), and conventional pulmonary digital subtraction angiography (**c**) for the right pulmonary artery (A10) in a 72-year-old woman with CTEPH. This data is quoted from the reference No. 8

monary artery collateral supply, distal to the CTO of the left inferior pulmonary artery trunk [6]. They concluded that 4D CTA can support embolization for systemic artery-to-pulmonary artery collaterals and to challenge BPA for a CTO lesion by identifying more distal vessel structures, including a retrograde approach. Although this is a more advanced technique for BPA operators who have recently started the procedure, their report may expand the potential of CT to guide BPA. Taken together, it seems to be not enough in a current practice only to perform conventional CTPA and pulmonary DSA before starting a BPA procedure, and we need to obtain sufficient information about web formation and distal vessel

structures up to subsegmental arteries using high-quality CT, which may lead to a lower dose of contrast agent, less radiation exposure, and perhaps less complications related to BPA.

8.3 Previously Published Noninvasive Imaging Technique to Evaluate BPA Efficacy

There have also been a lot of publications related to noninvasive imaging technique to evaluate BPA efficacy, including echocardiography, CT, and CMR. In this section, we focus on the recent

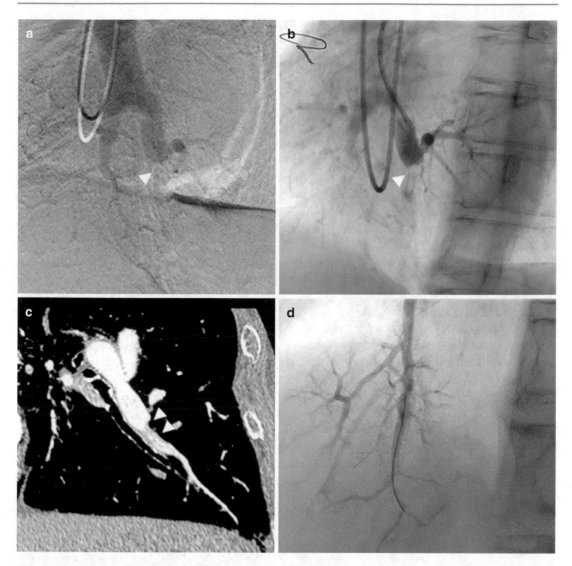

Fig. 8.3 Comparison of electrocardiogram-gated area detector computed tomography (ADCT) for target lesion assessment with conventional pulmonary digital subtraction angiography (DSA) and selective angiography during balloon pulmonary angioplasty (BPA). Representative image of DSA (**a**), selective angiography during BPA (**b**), ADCT image (**c**), and selective angiography after a successful BPA procedure (**d**) for the right pulmonary artery (A10) in a patient with chronic thromboembolic pulmonary hypertension. This data is quoted from the reference No. 11

publications related to CMR. In 2014, we published a study demonstrating right ventricular (RV) reverse remodeling, using cine CMR, after a series of BPA [13]. Right-heart function is considered to be one of the strong predictors of outcomes in CTEPH and, in that report, in all patients RV dilatation, dysfunction, hypertro-phy, and interventricular septal bowing were improved after BPA, differently from left ventricular (LV) function that remained unchanged. However, in 2016, Sato et al. from our group reported that a series of BPA significantly improved both RV and LV function [14]. In 2015, Ota et al., again from our CTEPH team, reported the successful visualization of drastic changes in vortex flow in the main pulmonary artery after a series of BPA using 4D flow CMR [15]. Kamada and Ota et al. also demonstrated in 2020 that 4D flow CMR detected the change in the volume flow rates of pulmonary arteries in a patient with suspected Takayasu's arteritis and isolated pulmonary artery involvement complicated with severe pulmonary hypertension (PH), where stent placement for stenosis in the right main pulmonary artery resulted in an increase in overall pulmonary blood flow and also improved blood flow balance between the right and left pulmonary arteries, with improved mean pulmonary arterial pressure from 45 to 22 mmHg [16]. Their work is worthy of note because they proposed direct assessment of pulmonary flow as a measure of efficacy of BPA with 4D flow CMR, whereas cine CMR indirectly assesses BPA efficacy by targeting cardiac function, but not pulmonary flow. In 2020, Yamasaki et al. demonstrated in 29 CTEPH patients that RA function such as the RA reservoir and passive conduit function significantly improved after a series of BPA, which was evaluated with cine CMR and a feature-tracking algorithm [17]. Thus, they successfully expand the target in efficacy evaluation after BPA using CMR, from RV function and pulmonary flow to RA function.

8.4 Current Practice Before and During a BPA Procedure in Our CTEPH Team

In the current practice of our CTEPH team, we consider CTPA as the best navigator for the successful BPA. In our institution, all patients without allergy to iodinated contrast agents undergo CTPA with ultrahigh-resolution CT (Aquilion Precision; Canon Medical Systems), which provides 0.25 mm-in-plane and z-axis resolution of the pulmonary artery. The high-resolution CT images visualize the morphology of lesions, vessel diameter, and vessel running direction in the pulmonary arteries up to at least subsegmental arteries (Fig. 8.4). 3D volume rendering (VR) images of the CTPA provide overview of the anatomy of pulmonary arteries and location of the legions. In addition, regional pulmonary blood distribution is evaluated from lung subtraction iodine maps, which are generated by subtraction of non-contrast images from CTPA images. "Iodine map," generalized by dualenergy or spectral CT, can also demonstrate the distribution of lung blood volume. Thus, a main operator (PH physician) of BPA determines targeted vessels or lesions the day before a BPA procedure, in subsequent discussion with experienced interventional radiologists, who finally determine the selection of suitable guiding cath-

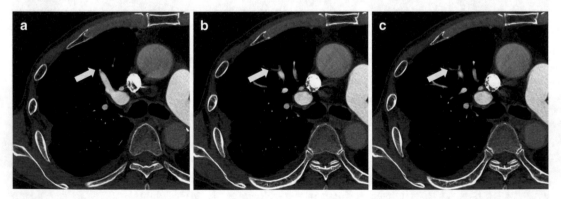

Fig. 8.4 High-quality image obtained from very thin slice of computed tomography in our hospital. Representative image of very thin slice of 0.25 mm of contrast-enhanced CT (**a–c**) for the right pulmonary artery (A3) in a patient with chronic thromboembolic pulmonary hypertension who underwent balloon pulmonary angioplasty. Note: There is abrupt narrowing in the bifurcation into subsegmental level of right A3 due to the web formation (*arrow*)

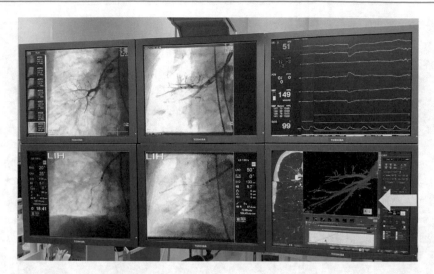

Fig. 8.5 Three-dimensional image of computed tomography (CT) monitored during a balloon pulmonary angioplasty procedure in our hospital. Three-dimensional (3D) image of CT (*arrow*) monitored and set up at the same angle as a projection angle, next to ongoing angiographical image with a biplane setting, in treating the right pulmonary artery (A4) in a patient with chronic thromboembolic pulmonary hypertension. Note: We can continuously confirm the position of a tip of a guide wire or a guiding catheter by referring to this 3D image, which can be rotated 360 degrees (*arrow*)

eter and projection angle in the session. During a BPA procedure, we can continuously confirm the position of the tip of a guide wire or a guiding catheter by referring to 3D VR monitored and set up at the same angle as a projection angle, next to ongoing angiographical image (Fig. 8.5). Also, we easily distinguish the most suitable projection angle by rotating the 3D image of CT 360 degrees (Fig. 8.5). Because we do not routinely use IVUS during BPA, we determine the appropriate size of a balloon, mainly based upon a diameter measured by CT.

When we look for a CTO in preparation before BPA, we adjust window settings of CT images from the mediastinal to the lung window to visualize peripheral branches of occluded pulmonary arteries from the bronchial tubes that normally run in along with the arteries. If a large bronchial tube is running alone, we consider the possibility that a relatively large CTO exists around the area (Fig. 8.6).

In rare cases with a history of significant allergy against contrast agent such as anaphylactic shock, we perform gadolinium-enhancement magnetic resonance imaging to evaluate the distribution of web formation and vessel stenosis/obstruction up to probably proximal segmental arteries. Then, we assess the operability of PEA and recommend PEA to a patient unless he/she has distal, surgically inaccessible thrombi or significant small-vessel arteriopathy. However, we consider BPA using CO_2 as the negative contrast agent for a patient who flatly refused PEA or has more distal-type disease. In such a rare case with CO_2, we cannot obtain clear image with selective angiography alone, and therefore we use IVUS to obtain intravascular imaging such as organized thrombi and vessel diameter.

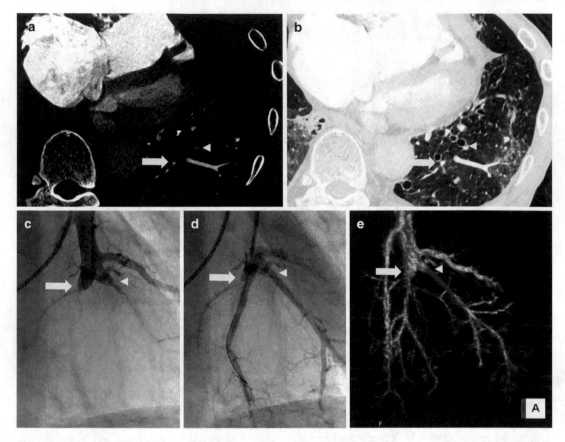

Fig. 8.6 Balloon pulmonary angioplasty (BPA) for a chronic total occlusion (CTO) using the lung window view of computed tomography (CT). Representative image of the mediastinal (**a**) and the lung window (**b**) view of thin-slice CT with corresponding angiographical image (**c, d**) for the left pulmonary artery (A9 *arrowhead* and A10 *arrow*) in a patient with chronic thromboembolic pulmonary hypertension. We successfully performed BPA for this CTO and subtotal lesions by referring to a three-dimensional vascular tree (**e**), which is reconstructed and clearly shows vessel diameter and vessel running direction at more distal portion than CTO lesions, even before starting BPA. Note: In panel B, A9 and A10 are running in along with the large bronchial tubes, although we could not conclude these vessels to be arteries or veins from panel A alone

8.5 Conclusions

In current practice, we need high-quality CT and its evaluation by the multidisciplinary CTEPH team, besides conventional CTPA and pulmonary DSA, before starting a BPA procedure, which may lead to a lower dose of contrast agent, less radiation exposure, and probably less complications related to BPA.

Acknowledgements We are very grateful to Mitsuru Nakada for his technical assistance for BPA procedures in our CTEPH team.

References

1. Feinstein JA, Goldhaber SZ, Lock JE, Ferndandes SM, Landzberg MJ. Balloon pulmonary angioplasty for treatment of chronic thromboembolic pulmonary hypertension. Circulation. 2001;103(1):10–3.
2. Mizoguchi H, Ogawa A, Munemasa M, Mikouchi H, Ito H, Matsubara H. Refined balloon pulmonary angioplasty for inoperable patients with chronic thromboembolic pulmonary hypertension. Circ Cardiovasc Interv. 2012;5(6):748–55.
3. Inami T, Kataoka M, Shimura N, Ishiguro H, Yanagisawa R, Fukuda K, Yoshino H, Satoh T. Pressure-wire-guided percutaneous transluminal pulmonary angioplasty: a breakthrough in catheter-

interventional therapy for chronic thromboembolic pulmonary hypertension. JACC Cardiovasc Interv. 2014;7(11):1297–306.

4. Sugimura K, Fukumoto Y, Miura Y, Nochioka K, Miura M, Tatebe S, Aoki T, Satoh K, Yamamoto S, Yaoita N, et al. Three-dimensional-optical coherence tomography imaging of chronic thromboembolic pulmonary hypertension. Eur Heart J. 2013;34(28):2121.

5. Lin JL, Chen HM, Lin FC, Li JY, Xie CX, Guo WL, Huang XF, Hong C. Application of DynaCT angiographic reconstruction in balloon pulmonary angioplasty. Eur Radiol. 2020;30:6950–7.

6. Tamura M, Kawakami T, Yamada Y, Kataoka M, Nakatsuka S, Fukuda K, Jinzaki M. Successful depiction of systemic collateral supply to pulmonary artery in CTEPH using time-resolved 4D CT angiography: a case report. Pulm Circ. 2020;10(2):2045894019881065.

7. Sugiyama M, Fukuda T, Sanda Y, Morita Y, Higashi M, Ogo T, Tsuji A, Demachi J, Nakanishi N, Naito H. Organized thrombus in pulmonary arteries in patients with chronic thromboembolic pulmonary hypertension; imaging with cone beam computed tomography. Jpn J Radiol. 2014;32(7):375–82.

8. Fukuda T, Ogo T, Nakanishi N, Ueda J, Sanda Y, Morita Y, Sugiyama M, Fukui S, Tsuji A, Naito H. Evaluation of organized thrombus in distal pulmonary arteries in patients with chronic thromboembolic pulmonary hypertension using cone-beam computed tomography. Jpn J Radiol. 2016;34(6):423–31.

9. Hinrichs JB, Marquardt S, von Falck C, Hoeper MM, Olsson KM, Wacker FK, Meyer BC. Comparison of C-arm computed tomography and digital subtraction angiography in patients with chronic thromboembolic pulmonary hypertension. Cardiovasc Intervent Radiol. 2016;39(1):53–63.

10. Hinrichs JB, Renne J, Hoeper MM, Olsson KM, Wacker FK, Meyer BC. Balloon pulmonary angioplasty: applicability of C-arm CT for procedure guidance. Eur Radiol. 2016;26(11):4064–71.

11. Ogo T, Fukuda T, Tsuji A, Fukui S, Ueda J, Sanda Y, Morita Y, Asano R, Konagai N, Yasuda S. Efficacy and safety of balloon pulmonary angioplasty for chronic thromboembolic pulmonary hypertension guided by cone-beam computed tomography and

electrocardiogram-gated area detector computed tomography. Eur J Radiol. 2017;89:270–6.

12. Takagi H, Ota H, Sugimura K, Otani K, Tominaga J, Aoki T, Tatebe S, Miura M, Yamamoto S, Sato H, et al. Dual-energy CT to estimate clinical severity of chronic thromboembolic pulmonary hypertension: comparison with invasive right heart catheterization. Eur J Radiol. 2016;85(9):1574–80.

13. Fukui S, Ogo T, Morita Y, Tsuji A, Tateishi E, Ozaki K, Sanda Y, Fukuda T, Yasuda S, Ogawa H, et al. Right ventricular reverse remodelling after balloon pulmonary angioplasty. Eur Respir J. 2014;43(5):1394–402.

14. Sato H, Ota H, Sugimura K, Aoki T, Tatebe S, Miura M, Yamamoto S, Yaoita N, Suzuki H, Satoh K, et al. Balloon pulmonary angioplasty improves biventricular functions and pulmonary flow in chronic thromboembolic pulmonary hypertension. Circ J. 2016;80(6):1470–7.

15. Ota H, Sugimura K, Miura M, Shimokawa H. Four-dimensional flow magnetic resonance imaging visualizes drastic change in vortex flow in the main pulmonary artery after percutaneous transluminal pulmonary angioplasty in a patient with chronic thromboembolic pulmonary hypertension. Eur Heart J. 2015;36(25):1630.

16. Kamada H, Ota H, Aoki T, Sugimura K, Yaoita N, Shimokawa H, Takase K. 4D-flow MRI assessment of blood flow before and after endovascular intervention in a patient with pulmonary hypertension due to isolated pulmonary artery involvement in large vessel vasculitis. Radiol Case Rep. 2020;15(3):190–4.

17. Yamasaki Y, Abe K, Kamitani T, Hosokawa K, Kawakubo M, Sagiyama K, Hida T, Matsuura Y, Murayama Y, Funatsu R, et al. Balloon pulmonary angioplasty improves right atrial reservoir and conduit functions in chronic thromboembolic pulmonary hypertension. Eur Heart J Cardiovasc Imaging. 2020;21(8):855–62.

18. Maschke SK, Hinrichs JB, Renne J, Werncke T, Winther HMB, Ringe KI, Olsson KM, Hoeper MM, Wacker FK, Meyer BC. C-arm computed tomography (CACT)-guided balloon pulmonary angioplasty (BPA): evaluation of patient safety and peri- and post-procedural complications. Eur Radiol. 2019;29(3):1276–84.

Hiroto Shimokawahara, Aiko Ogawa,
and Hiromi Matsubara

9.1 Introduction

Pulmonary endarterectomy (PEA) [1–3] remains the treatment of choice for patients with chronic thromboembolic pulmonary hypertension (CTEPH). However, even though the lesions are surgically accessible and suitable for PEA, some patients could not be candidates for PEA. Patients with advanced age, comorbidities, or poor general condition are considered ineligible for PEA [4], because PEA is an invasive procedure generally performed under intermittent total circulatory arrest with deep hypothermia [1–3]. Thus, an alternative treatment option might be appropriate. Balloon pulmonary angioplasty (BPA) is a promising therapeutic option for patients with CTEPH who are ineligible for PEA [5–8]. However, while treatment with BPA of distal

lesions in segmental and subsegmental pulmonary arteries is widely performed and accepted, proximal lesions that should be treated with PEA are considered unsuitable for BPA. It remains unclear whether BPA would become an alternative treatment for patients with proximal lesions who cannot be candidates for PEA. We will summarize the effectiveness of BPA in proximal lesions based on previous reports and our own experiences. Additionally, we will address the limitations and future perspectives of BPA in proximal lesions.

9.2 Therapeutic Outcomes of BPA in Proximal Lesions

Because there is no strict definition of proximal lesions with CTEPH on angiography, the proximal lesions in this chapter are defined as those with thrombi starting at the level of the lobar arteries or main descending pulmonary arteries. Previously, patients with proximal lesions had been considered out of indication for BPA because of concerns regarding the decreased effectiveness of BPA and the high risk of complications in these patients. In particular, treating total occlusion lesions in proximal pulmonary arteries by BPA has been thought to be a contraindication because of the danger of potentially fatal reperfusion pulmonary edema [9]. With the rapidly increasing experience in BPA expert cen-

H. Shimokawahara (✉)
Department of Cardiology, National Hospital Organization Okayama Medical Center, Okayama, Japan

A. Ogawa
Department of Clinical Science, National Hospital Organization Okayama Medical Center, Okayama, Japan

H. Matsubara
Department of Cardiology, National Hospital Organization Okayama Medical Center, Okayama, Japan

Department of Clinical Science, National Hospital Organization Okayama Medical Center, Okayama, Japan

© Springer Nature Switzerland AG 2022
F. Saia et al. (eds.), *Balloon pulmonary angioplasty in patients with CTEPH*,
https://doi.org/10.1007/978-3-030-95997-5_9

ters, BPA is becoming a therapeutic option for inoperable CTEPH patients with proximal lesions. Nevertheless, previous reports demonstrating the outcome of BPA in proximal lesions are only a few case reports or case series [10, 11]. According to our experience, among 345 CTEPH patients treated with BPA in our hospital, 23% had proximal lesions. The improvements in hemodynamics obtained by BPA in these patients were not inferior compared to those in other patients who only had distal lesions. In addition, the cumulative survival rate was not different between the two groups [12]. However, in this study, patients with proximal lesions were also treated for distal lesions with BPA at the same time. No other data are available to show the outcome of BPA treating only proximal lesions.

9.3   General BPA Procedure

The general BPA procedure for proximal lesions is essentially the same as that for distal lesions. The basic BPA technique in our hospital is described in detail in Chap. 5. We have previously reported that both the success rate and complication rate vary across angiographical lesion types (ringlike stenosis, web lesions, subtotal occlusion lesions, total occlusion lesions, and tortuous lesions) [13]. In particular, the success rate of BPA highly depends on whether the lesions are totally occluded or not. This result seems to be more prominent in proximal lesions. Conversely, web lesions and tortuous lesions are rarely observed within proximal lesions. Therefore, in this chapter, we focus on the specialized techniques of BPA for proximal lesions and illustrate the tips and tricks of BPA in ringlike stenosis, subtotal occlusion lesions, and total occlusion lesions.

9.4   Basic Techniques for Proximal Lesions

9.4.1   Approach and Selection of the Guiding Catheter

We usually perform BPA through the right femoral vein because one operator can manipulate both the guiding catheter and guidewire with lower radiation exposure compared to the right jugular vein approach. In contrast, the right jugular vein approach is useful in treating total occlusion lesions with hard fibrous tissue in the right lung because a strong backup force can be obtained. For lesions requiring stronger backup force, a 7–8-Fr guiding catheter with a 7–8-Fr-long introducer sheath (BRITE TIP® Sheath Introducer; Cordis, Santa Clara, California, USA) should be selected. However, it is difficult to manipulate large-profile guiding catheters in the right ventricle or pulmonary artery. We frequently use a 4-Fr Judkins Right-4 diagnostic catheter as a daughter catheter in such cases. The most important determinant to increase the success rate of treating proximal total occlusion lesions is the selection of the shape of the guiding catheter. Currently, there are no guiding catheters specialized for BPA. We usually select the guiding catheter for the peripheral or coronary artery, such as the Mach 1 peripheral MP for the bilateral lower and upper lobes and a Mach 1 AL1 catheter for the right middle lobe and lingula lobe. The Mach 1 Q-Curve (Boston Scientific, Marlborough, MA, USA) is also useful when a strong-edged curve of the guiding catheter is necessary. In addition, we usually adjust the shape of the guiding catheter by advancing or pulling back the long sheath if these catheters do not align coaxially to the lesion.

9.4.2   Lesion Dilation for Proximal Lesions

It is necessary to determine how much to dilate the lesion to achieve maximal therapeutic efficacy while reducing the risk of pulmonary vessel injury. The balloon size should be decided based on the original vessel diameter, the amount of fibrous tissues at the lesions, and the hemodynamics of each patient [14]. In the current strategy of BPA for distal lesions, we dilate the lesions with a 2.0 mm balloon in the initial treatment. Then, 1–3 months after the initial dilation, repeat dilation of the same lesions with appropriate balloon diameters (3.0–6.0 mm) is performed to finalize the intervention [15]. In the treatment of proximal lesions, it is also essential to dilate the lesions sequentially in a stepwise manner. However, a 2.0 mm balloon is too small to dilate the proximal lesions, even in the initial BPA procedure, to maintain the patency of the lesions at the following BPA procedure. The original vessel diameters in the proximal lesions are much larger than those in the distal lesions. A larger balloon size should be selected based on the vessel diameter just proximal to the lesion not only in the initial BPA procedure but also in the secondary dilation to optimize the result. If it is difficult to select the balloon size based only on pulmonary angiography, the use of intravascular ultrasound (IVUS) should be considered. The adequate balloon size for each thromboembolic lesion type is described below.

9.4.3 Tips and Tricks Based on Angiographical Lesion Types

9.4.3.1 Ringlike Stenosis
In distal lesions, the success rate of BPA for ringlike stenosis is much higher than that for other lesion types [13]. Passing the guidewire through the lesion is not so complicated that it is important to select a guidewire with the smallest possible tip load to reduce the risk of vessel injury caused by the guidewire. The only essential tip for the treatment of ringlike stenosis is the selection of the balloon size. Because this type of lesion easily recoils due to circumferential elastic

hard fibrous tissues, a bigger balloon size (120–150% of the reference vessel diameter) should be selected to obtain maximum lumen enlargement. The use of a scoring balloon or buddy wire is an option if the balloon catheter easily slips distal or proximal to the lesion. The use of a cutting balloon is not recommended because of the high risk of vessel injury.

Figure 9.1 shows the representative pulmonary angiography images before (Fig. 9.1a) and after BPA (Fig. 9.1b) in a 66-year-old female patient with proximal ringlike stenoses. She refused PEA, so we had to treat her with BPA. Since the mean pulmonary arterial pressure (PAP) before BPA was less than 40 mmHg, we selected a larger balloon size relative to the actual vessel diameter (4.0–6.0 mm balloon) from the initial BPA procedure. After only two BPA procedures, the mean PAP decreased from 36 mmHg to 18 mmHg, and the pulmonary vascular resistance (PVR) decreased from 7.5 wood units to 3.3 wood units.

9.4.3.2 Subtotal Occlusion Lesions
Figure 9.2 shows the representative pulmonary angiography images before (Fig. 9.2a) and after BPA (Fig. 9.2b) in an 81-year-old female patient with proximal subtotal occlusion lesions, particularly in the right lung. Although according to the findings of pulmonary angiography before BPA (Fig. 9.2a) the patient appeared to be a good candidate for PEA, she was considered inoperable because of her advanced age. Selective pulmo-

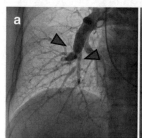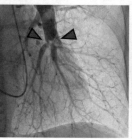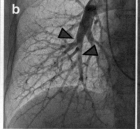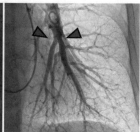

Fig. 9.1 Representative global pulmonary angiography image in a patient with chronic thromboembolic pulmonary hypertension (CTEPH) with ringlike stenoses at the proximal site. (**a**) Global pulmonary angiography image before balloon pulmonary angioplasty (BPA). Ringlike stenoses (red arrow) were observed in the lower lobar

arteries in both lungs. Pulmonary vessels distal to the lesions were observed with shrinkage. (**b**) Global pulmonary angiography after BPA. The treated lesions, including pulmonary vessels distal to the lesions, were enlarged after two BPA procedures

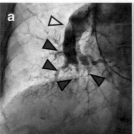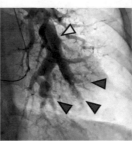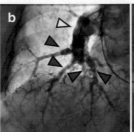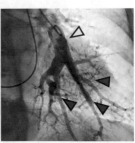

Fig. 9.2 Representative global pulmonary angiography image in a patient with chronic thromboembolic pulmonary hypertension (CTEPH) with subtotal occlusion lesions at the proximal sites. (**a**) Global pulmonary angiography image before BPA. Severe stenoses (red arrow) in the right lung were observed, and pulmonary arteries distal to the lesions were not visible in some portions. Subtotal occlusions at the middle portion of the segmental pulmonary arteries in the left lobe were also observed. The bilateral main descending pulmonary arteries are enlarged (yellow arrow). (**b**) After BPA. The lesions and pulmonary vessels distal to the lesions were enlarged after eight BPA procedures despite the remaining irregularities of the pulmonary arterial wall. Bilateral enlargement of the main descending pulmonary arteries became smaller after BPA (yellow arrow)

nary angiography displays many collateral vessels toward the total or subtotal occlusion sites in other segmental pulmonary arteries (Fig. 9.3a, b). Obstructions distal to the subsegmental arteries with a vessel size of 2–3 mm are hard to detect prior to PEA, especially in patients with proximal lesions. These vessel abnormalities in distal lesions mixed with proximal lesions might be one of the reasons for residual pulmonary hypertension after PEA. After eight BPA procedures in this case, the mean PAP decreased from 51 mmHg to 27 mmHg, and the PVR decreased from 12.8 wood units to 4.3 wood units.

The success of BPA for subtotal occlusion lesions highly depends on whether the guidewire can be passed through the lesion and select the true lumen of the distal vessels. Thus, it is essential to obtain as much information regarding vessels distal to the occluded lesions as possible before trying to pass the lesions with a guidewire. Make sure to properly perform selective pulmonary angiography, injecting a diluted contrast with saline at adequate pressure with maximum inspiration. Conducting selective pulmonary angiography using 8-inch images similar to a coronary intervention is also essential to obtain precise distal information. Even though the lesion appears to be totally occluded (Fig. 9.3c), it is often possible to detect the microchannel by placing the guiding catheter coaxially close to the occluded site, as indicated in Fig. 9.3d. This lesion was dilated with a 2.0 mm balloon after successfully passing the guidewire through the lesion (Fig. 9.3e).

The operator should advance the guidewire in a sliding manner to avoid entering a false channel without pushing the guidewire excessively at the beginning. Advancing the guidewire via a false channel could result in pulmonary artery dissection, which can lead to reocclusion of the treated site as well as reduce the success rate. The guidewire should be pulled back a little and advanced in the other direction to enter the correct microchannel if the guidewire is stuck within the lesion even though the distal channel is visible on pulmonary angiography. In addition, if the guiding catheter is moving due to breathing or heartbeats, it is not easy to advance the guidewire. Therefore, it is essential to stabilize the guiding catheter at the same position to treat subtotal occlusion lesions at the proximal site. We usually advance the guidewire during maximum inspiration when the pulmonary arteries are straightening. It facilitates the passage of the guidewire through the lesions. Although it is ideal to use a guidewire with the smallest possible tip load, using a microcatheter or other guidewires with a heavier tip load (a tip load ≤3 g would be sufficient in most cases) should be considered if soft-tip guidewires cannot pass the lesions. After successfully passing the guidewire through the lesion, it is necessary to change the guidewire to a soft-tip one

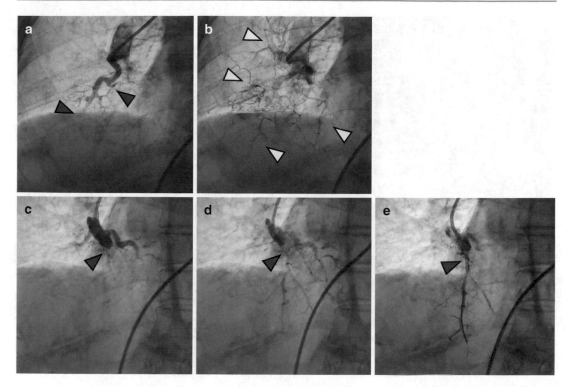

Fig. 9.3 Fluoroscopic images before, during, and immediately after balloon pulmonary angioplasty (BPA) in the first BPA procedure. (**a**) Selective pulmonary angiography image of the lateral basal segmental artery of the right lower lobe (A9). Pulmonary arteries distal to the subsegmental pulmonary arteries were not visible in some portions (red arrow). (**b**) Many collateral vessels toward the other totally occluded lesions became visible after a short period of selective pulmonary angiography of the right A9 (yellow arrow). (**c**) Selective pulmonary angiography of the posterior basal segmental artery of the right lower lobe (A10). It appears totally occluded (red arrow). (**d**) Selective pulmonary angiography of the right A10 after placing the guiding catheter close to the occlusion site and adjusting the guiding catheter coaxially. The distal vessel became visible (red arrow). (**e**) Selective pulmonary angiography image after dilating the lesion with a 2.0 mm balloon. The lesion and distal vessels were enlarged after balloon dilation (red arrow)

using a microcatheter in case of utilizing a guidewire with a tip load ≥2 g. Before dilation of the lesion, it is necessary to confirm whether the guidewire is in the correct microchannel by checking the pulmonary angiography or IVUS results.

When dilating subtotal occlusion lesions at the proximal site, much attention should be paid to select the balloon size because of the difference in the lumen size at the lesion and the lesion proximal vessel. In the initial BPA procedure, we usually select the balloon 60–80% of the reference vessel diameter and only dilate the critical site without dilating the distal lesions. In the following BPA procedure, we dilate the lesion again with an optimized size balloon and treat the distal lesion if necessary.

9.4.3.3 Total Occlusion Lesions

Total occlusion lesions existing at the proximal segmental pulmonary arteries or more proximal pulmonary arteries are completely different from those existing at the subsegmental pulmonary arteries. Usually, the appearance of these lesions is a typical "pouch." Pulmonary angiography findings in a 57-year-old female patient with a total occlusion lesion in the lower lobar artery of the right lung showed that the lesion was totally covered by the intima, and its surface was smooth (Fig. 9.4a). There was no trace of the vessels distal to the lesion. The lesion itself consists of 2–4 layers of extremely hard fibrous tissues and rough fibrous tissues filling between each hard layer. Even with an extremely hard-tip wire with more than a 10 g tip load,

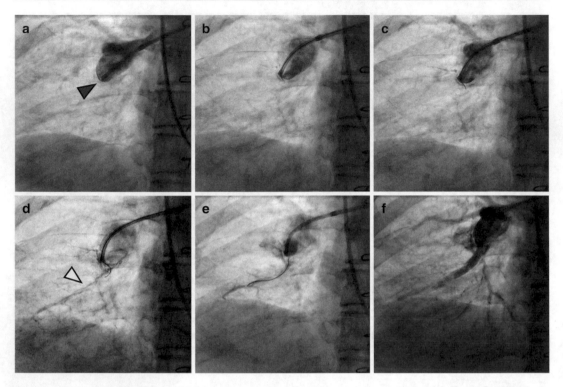

Fig. 9.4 Fluoroscopic images before, during, and immediately after balloon pulmonary angioplasty (BPA) for total occlusion lesion of the right lower lobar artery. (**a**) The right lower lobar artery was totally occluded with a smooth surface (red arrow). (**b**) The guidewire did not advance because of the hard layer at the occlusion site. (**c**) Advancing the guidewire little by little by deliberately dissecting the intima at the lesion upon contacting the tip of the guiding catheter to the lesion and injecting a small amount of contrast medium. (**d**) Advancing the hard-tip wire with a microcatheter into the space caused by the dissection to penetrate the first hard layer. The distal vessel became visible on repeated pulmonary angiography (yellow arrow). (**e**) Even after passing the lesion by a guidewire, information of the distal vessels is difficult to obtain. Before dilating the lesion, the guidewire should be changed to a soft tip using a microcatheter and confirm the position of the guidewire using intravascular ultrasound. (**f**) Final selective pulmonary angiography in the first BPA procedure after sequential dilation with a 3.0 and 6.0 mm balloon

which is used for penetration of the total occlusion lesions in peripheral arteries, penetration of the first hard layer would not be possible. In such cases, the first step is to deliberately dissect the intima at the lesion by contacting the tip of the guiding catheter to the lesion and injecting a small amount of contrast medium (Fig. 9.4b). The second step is to proceed with the hard-tip wire with a microcatheter into the space caused by dissection to penetrate the first hard layer. After penetrating the first hard layer, the first step should be repeated to create another dissection under the first layer. Then, procedures should be repeated until the guidewire can penetrate the final hard layer (Fig. 9.4c, d).

During the procedure, repeated angiography may offer information distal to the lesion. Usually, however, even after passing the lesion by the guidewire, information of distal vessels is difficult to obtain (Fig. 9.4e). Thus, the use of IVUS is necessary in most cases to confirm the guidewire position. If the guidewire is outside the vessels, pulling back the guidewire is sufficient to prevent bleeding. The lesion contains a large amount of fibrous tissues and can easily fill the pin hall made by wire perforation. The procedure can be continued after pulling back the guidewire. If the guidewire is inside the vessels, it should be changed to the soft-tip wire using a microcatheter because the vessels distal

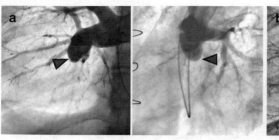
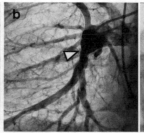
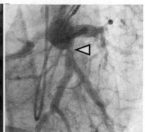
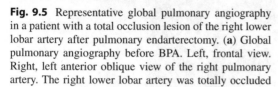

Fig. 9.5 Representative global pulmonary angiography in a patient with a total occlusion lesion of the right lower lobar artery after pulmonary endarterectomy. (**a**) Global pulmonary angiography before BPA. Left, frontal view. Right, left anterior oblique view of the right pulmonary artery. The right lower lobar artery was totally occluded with a smooth surface (red arrow). (**b**) Global pulmonary angiography after BPA. Left, frontal view. Right, left anterior oblique view of the right pulmonary artery. The lesion has maintained patency for nine years despite the remaining irregularities of the pulmonary arterial wall at the occluded site (yellow arrow)

to the total occlusion lesions are usually very fragile and easily injured by a hard-tip wire. After sequential dilation with a 3.0 and 6.0 mm balloon, the BPA procedure could be completed (Fig. 9.4f).

Figure 9.5 shows the representative pulmonary angiography images before (Fig. 9.5a) and after BPA (Fig. 9.5b) with a total occlusion lesion in the lower lobar artery of the right lung, the same patient as indicated in Fig. 9.4. The occlusion site, which was treated 9 years ago, is still patent. The mean PAP, which had been elevated even after PEA, decreased from 36 mmHg to 18 mmHg after seven BPA procedures. The PVR was also reduced from 7.5 wood units to 3.3 wood units.

Generally, it would be impossible to complete the treatment for proximal total occlusion lesions with only a single BPA procedure. Total occlusion lesions should be treated sequentially in several separate procedures, not only to reduce the occurrence of vessel injury but also to increase the success rate. In the initial BPA procedure, it is essential to terminate the procedure by restoring the minimum blood flow through the lesion to maintain the lesion patency until the following BPA procedure. It is important to open a few branches if possible, to maintain blood flow. If the treated lesion maintains patency, spontaneous enlargement of the treated site, including distal vessels, can be expected, as in the distal lesions. Occasionally, some occluded branches would become visible spontaneously. Additional dilation of the occluded site using the optimal bal-

loon size, treating the distal lesions, and treating other newly visualized branches are the main purposes of the next BPA procedure.

Figure 9.6 shows another representative BPA procedure for a 63-year-old patient with a total occlusion lesion at the lower lobar artery of the right lung (Fig. 9.6a). After crossing the guidewire through the fibrous cap and dilating the lesion with a 5.0 mm balloon (Fig. 9.6b), the second total occlusion lesion existing at the distal to the first occluded site was recognized (Fig. 9.6c). After treating three branches at the second occluded site, the blood flow dramatically improved (Fig. 9.6d). Treating more distal lesions, such as distal to subsegmental pulmonary arteries, should be avoided during the first BPA procedure for the treatment of total occlusion lesions because of the fragility of the distal vessels.

Because of the large amounts of fibrous tissues, including hard layers, balloon dilation of the total occlusion lesions is different from other lesion types. Using smaller balloons compared to the original vessel diameter frequently resulted in reocclusion of the lesions, probably because of recoil. Dilation with sufficiently large balloons without causing vessel injury is necessary to maintain patency at the lesion. One month after the initial BPA procedure, residual stenoses remained at the previously occluded site (Fig. 9.6e). After dilating the lesion with a 10 mm balloon (Fig. 9.6f), the occluded site and the vessels distal to the lesions were further enlarged (Fig. 9.6g). Considering the complexity of this

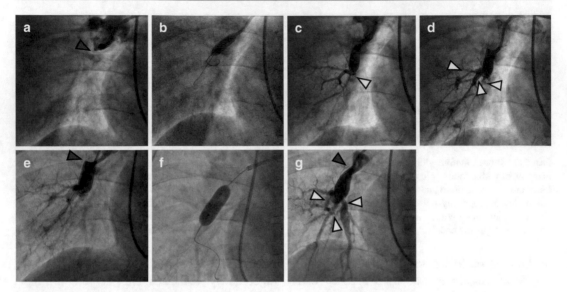

Fig. 9.6 Fluoroscopic images before and immediately after balloon pulmonary angioplasty (BPA) for total occlusion lesion of the right lower lobe in the first and second BPA procedures. (**a**) The right lower lobar artery was totally occluded (red arrow). (**b**) After crossing the guidewire through the first fibrous cap and dilating the lesion with a 5.0 mm balloon. (**c**) Selective pulmonary angiography after dilation of the first occluded site. The second occluded site distal to the first occluded site became visible (yellow arrow). (**d**) Final selective pulmo-nary angiography in the first BPA procedure after treating three branches (yellow arrow) at the second occluded site. (**e**) Selective pulmonary angiography in the second BPA procedure. Residual stenosis remained at the first occluded site (red arrow). (**f**) Dilation of the residual stenotic lesion with a 10 mm balloon. (**g**) Final selective pulmonary angiography in the second BPA procedure. Both the first occluded site (red arrow) and the second occluded site (yellow arrow) enlarged after balloon dilation

procedure and the high risk of complications, treatment of proximally existing total occlusion lesions should be considered at the final phase of BPA treatment in each patient. In addition, it should be performed by highly experienced BPA operators. In our previous report, the success rate of BPA for total occlusion lesions was 52.2%, which was extremely lower than that for other lesion types [13]. Since the success rate included the treatment for distal lesions, it might have been even lower when limited to the treatment for proximal lesions. In our recent preliminary data, the success rate of BPA for proximal total occlusion lesions was 79% whereas the patency rate at follow-up was only 59%.

9.5 Complications of BPA in Proximal Lesions

Even with maximum effort to avoid complications of BPA, it is impossible to eliminate their occurrence. The most frequent and characteristic complication of BPA is lung injury caused by vascular injury. There are no other specific complications of BPA in proximal lesions. However, lung injury tends to be exacerbated in BPA for proximal lesions. The treatment to stop bleeding at the injured site is more difficult in proximal lesions than in distal lesions. Temporary occlusion of the pulmonary artery by balloon inflation to stop bleeding at the proximal site is extremely difficult because of the large proximal pulmonary artery diameter. If bleeding occurs, neutralizing heparin and trying to occlude the proximal site of the lesion for 10–15 minutes with an adequate balloon size would be essential. When these procedures cannot control bleeding, an embolic agent should be injected into the injured vessel to seal the bleeding site. If bleeding cannot be controlled despite these efforts, usage of V-A extracorporeal membrane oxygenation should be considered. Endotracheal intubation and positive airway ventilation are usually not sufficient to stop bleeding because, in most cases, pulmonary artery pressure is much higher than airway pressure. In case of pulmonary artery rupture after balloon dilation, a covered stent can be a treatment option [16].

9.6 Limitations and Perspectives of BPA in Proximal Lesions

The efficacy and safety of BPA have improved dramatically in recent years (6.7.8). The effectiveness of BPA in patients with CTEPH who are ineligible for PEA despite having surgically accessible lesions might be acceptable compared with PEA. Thus, BPA might become an alternative treatment for such patients. However, a comparison of the therapeutic outcome of BPA between proximal and distal lesions has not yet been performed. BPA cannot resect fibrous tissues; therefore, the fibrous tissues at the lesion would be left permanently even after successful BPA procedures. This problem becomes more serious in proximal lesions than in distal lesions because of the larger amounts of fibrous tissues. Pulmonary angiography images after BPA in proximal lesions show irregularity of the proximal vessel wall, indicating the existence of the remaining fibrous tissues (Fig. 9.2b and 9.5b). So far, the only way to solve this problem is to dilate the lesion using oversize balloons while taking the risk of vessel injury. The effectiveness of stent implantation in proximal lesions has recently been reported [17]. Although stent implantation might be one of the solutions to maintain the patency of the proximal lesions after BPA, further studies are needed to clarify the safety, efficacy, and long-term patency.

9.7 Conclusions

Although the success rate and the follow-up patency rate of BPA for proximal total occlusion lesions appear to be lower, the therapeutic outcome of other lesion types in proximal lesions has dramatically improved. Further advances in therapeutic efficacy with minimal risk of complications could make BPA an alternative treatment option for not only CTEPH patients with distal lesions but also those with proximal lesions who are ineligible for PEA because of their comorbidities.

References

1. Madani MM, Auger WR, Pretorius V, Sakakibara N, Kerr KM, Kim NH, et al. Pulmonary endarterectomy: recent changes in a single institution's experience of more than 2,700 patients. Ann Thorac Surg. 2012;94:97–103. https://doi.org/10.1016/j.athoracsur.2012.04.004.
2. Jenkins D. Pulmonary endarterectomy: the potentially curative treatment for patients with chronic thromboembolic pulmonary hypertension. Eur Respir Rev. 2015;24:263–71. https://doi.org/10.1183/16000617.00000815.
3. Jenkins D, Madani M, Fadel E, D'Armini AM, Mayer E. Pulmonary endarterectomy in the management of chronic thromboembolic pulmonary hypertension. Eur Respir Rev. 2017;26:143. https://doi.org/10.1183/16000617.0111-2016.
4. Madani M, Mayer E, Fadel E, Jenkins DP. Pulmonary endarterectomy. Patient selection, technical challenges, and outcomes. Ann Am Thorac Soc. 2016;13:S240–7. https://doi.org/10.1513/AnnalsATS.201601-014AS.
5. Mizoguchi H, Ogawa A, Munemasa M, Mikouchi H, Ito H, Matsubara H. Refined balloon pulmonary angioplasty for inoperable patients with chronic thromboembolic pulmonary hypertension. Circ Cardiovasc Interv. 2012;5:748–55.
6. Ogawa A, Satoh T, Fukuda T, Sugimura K, Fukumoto Y, Emoto N, et al. Balloon pulmonary angioplasty for chronic thromboembolic pulmonary hypertension: results of a multicenter registry. Circ Cardiovasc Qual Outcomes. 2017;10:1. https://doi.org/10.1161/CIRCOUTCOMES.117.004029.
7. Lang I, Meyer BC, Ogo T, Matsubara H, Kurzyna M, Ghofrani HA, et al. Balloon pulmonary angioplasty in chronic thromboembolic pulmonary hypertension. Eur Respir Rev. 2017;2017:26. https://doi.org/10.1183/16000617.0119-2016.
8. Mahmud E, Madani MM, Kim NH, Poch D, Ang L, Behnamfar O, et al. Chronic thromboembolic pulmonary hypertension: evolving therapeutic approaches for operable and inoperable disease. J Am Coll Cardiol. 2018;71:2468–86. https://doi.org/10.1016/j.jacc.2018.04.009.
9. Feinstein JA, Goldhaber SZ, Lock JE, Ferndandes SM, Landzberg MJ. Balloon pulmonary angioplasty for treatment of chronic thromboembolic pulmonary hypertension. Circulation. 2001;103:10–3. https://doi.org/10.1161/01.CIR.103.1.10.
10. Minatsuki S, Kiyosue A, Kodera S, Hara T, Saito A, Maki H, et al. Effectiveness of balloon pulmonary angioplasty in patients with inoperable chronic thromboembolic pulmonary hypertension despite having lesion types suitable for surgical treatment.

J Cardiol. 2020;75:182–8. https://doi.org/10.1016/j.jjcc.2019.07.006.

11. Ishiguro H, Kataoka M, Inami T, Yanagisawa R, Shimura N, Taguchi H, et al. Percutaneous transluminal pulmonary angioplasty for central-type chronic thromboembolic pulmonary hypertension. JACC Cardiovasc Interv. 2013;6:1212–3. https://doi.org/10.1016/j.jcin.2013.03.025.

12. Nishihara T, Shimokawahara H, Matsubara H, Hayashi K, Tsuji M, Naito T, et al. The hemodynamic improvement with balloon pulmonary angioplasty in chronic thromboembolic pulmonary hypertension depends on the lesion location. Eur Heart J. 2019;40:1. https://doi.org/10.1093/eurheartj/ehz745.1060.

13. Kawakami T, Ogawa A, Miyaji K, Mizoguchi H, Shimokawahara H, Naito T, et al. Novel angiographic classification of each vascular lesion in chronic thromboembolic pulmonary hypertension based on selective angiogram and results of balloon pulmonary angioplasty. Circ Cardiovasc Interv. 2016;9:e003318. https://doi.org/10.1161/CIRCINTERVENTIONS.115.003318.

14. Shimokawahara H, Ogawa A, Mizoguchi H, Yagi H, Ikemiyagi H, Matsubara H. Vessel stretching is a cause of lumen enlargement immediately after balloon pulmonary angioplasty: intravascular ultrasound analysis in patients with chronic thromboembolic pulmonary hypertension. Circ Cardiovasc Interv. 2018;11:e006010. https://doi.org/10.1161/CIRCINTERVENTIONS.117.006010.

15. Ogawa A, Matsubara H. After the dawn—balloon pulmonary angioplasty for patients with chronic thromboembolic pulmonary hypertension. Circ J. 2018;82:1222–30. https://doi.org/10.1253/circj.CJ-18-0258.

16. Ejiri K, Ogawa A, Matsubara H. Bail-out technique for pulmonary artery rupture with a covered stent in balloon pulmonary angioplasty for chronic thromboembolic pulmonary hypertension. JACC Cardiovasc Interv. 2015;8:752–3. https://doi.org/10.1016/j.jcin.2014.11.024.

17. Darocha S, Pietura R, Banaszkiewicz M, Pietrasik A, Kownacki L, Torbicki A, et al. Balloon pulmonary angioplasty with stent implantation as a treatment of proximal chronic thromboembolic pulmonary hypertension. Diagnostics (Basel). 2020;10:6. https://doi.org/10.3390/diagnostics10060363.

Metrics for Success of Balloon Pulmonary Angioplasty in Chronic Thromboembolic Pulmonary Hypertension

Francesco Saia, Fabio Dardi, Nevio Taglieri, Alessandra Manes, Daniele Guarino, Nazzareno Galiè, and Massimiliano Palazzini

10.1 Introduction

The efficacy of a therapeutic intervention is measured through the assessment of its risk/benefit ratio. Balloon pulmonary angioplasty (BPA) in patients with chronic thromboembolic pulmonary hypertension (CTEPH) should not deviate from this general rule and rigorous scientific evaluation of its net clinical benefit is mandatory. Presently, BPA is still largely considered a compassionate procedure for symptomatic and inoperable patients and development of evidence is in the early phase. In this context, standardization of

definitions for outcomes of interest would be of the greatest importance in order to provide benchmark endpoints for BPA procedures and to improve interpretability and comparability of the results between different studies.

The efficacy of BPA to treat CTEPH could be measured with different perspectives, the principal being, of course, clinical outcomes. However, there are a number of surrogate endpoints that are known to correlate with the clinical outcome, such as changes in hemodynamics (e.g., reduction of pulmonary vascular resistance (PVR)) and right ventricular function (RV). Those patient-centered endpoints are often the result of multiple BPA procedures, each one targeting several lesions in different lung territories. Hence, physicians should also set parameters to evaluate the success of BPA at a lesion level, including residual stenosis, pulmonary vessel flow, and resting pressure gradient through the target lesion. All efficacy endpoints should then be weighed against safety, as measured by the occurrence of periprocedural complications.

The aim of this chapter is therefore to review endpoints and metrics commonly used in clinical practice and in scientific literature to define the success of BPA (Table 10.1).

F. Saia (✉) · N. Taglieri · A. Manes
Cardiology Unit, Cardio-Thoracic-Vascular Department, IRCCS University Hospital of Bologna, Policlinico S. Orsola, Bologna, Italy
e-mail: francesco.saia@unibo.it; nevio.taglieri@aosp.bo.it; alessandra.manes@unibo.it

F. Dardi · D. Guarino
Department of Experimental, Diagnostic and Specialty Medicine (DIMES), Bologna University Hospital, Bologna, Italy
e-mail: fabio.dardi@aosp.bo.it; daniele.guarino3@unibo.it

N. Galiè · M. Palazzini
Cardiology Unit, Cardio-Thoracic-Vascular Department, IRCCS University Hospital of Bologna, Policlinico S. Orsola, Bologna, Italy

Department of Experimental, Diagnostic and Specialty Medicine (DIMES), Bologna University Hospital, Bologna, Italy
e-mail: nazzareno.galie@unibo.it; massimiliano.palazzini@unibo.it

© Springer Nature Switzerland AG 2022
F. Saia et al. (eds.), *Balloon pulmonary angioplasty in patients with CTEPH*,
https://doi.org/10.1007/978-3-030-95997-5_10

Table 10.1 Treatment goals for balloon pulmonary angioplasty in CTEPH

	Parameter
Patient-level outcomes	
Clinical outcomes	
Increased survival	Relief of PH
Improved QoL	EQ-5D, CHAMPOR
Improved exercise capacity	6MWD, Borg, WHO
Symptom relief	Discontinuation or reduction of PH-specific drugs Discontinuation of home oxygen therapy Patient's preference (when patients believe that they no longer require additional BPA sessions)
Surrogate endpoints	
Relief of pulmonary hypertension	mPAP <25 mmHg mPAP <30 mmHg (alternative threshold used in many centers) PVR <3 wood units
Improved right ventricle (RV) function	Normalization of RV volume, ejection fraction, tricuspid annular plane systolic excursion (TAPSE), and RV free wall peak strain
Arterial oxygen saturation	>95%
Change in plasma brain natriuretic peptide levels	Normalization of BNP/NTpro-BNP
Target lesion endpoints	
Pulmonary flow grade[a]	=3
Pd/pa	>0.8
Procedural safety endpoints	
PEPSI[a]	<35
mPAP distal to treated lesion	<35 mm hg

PH pulmonary hypertension, *mPAP* mean pulmonary artery pressure, *Pd/Pa* ratio of distal:proximal pressures across the target lesion (detected by pressure wire), *PEPSI* pulmonary edema predictive scoring index, *PVR* pulmonary vascular resistance.

[a] as defined by Inami et al. [1]

10.2 Patient-Level Outcomes

10.2.1 Clinical Outcomes

Survival. CTEPH has a dramatic impact on the survival and quality of life, with important reduction of survival when mean pulmonary arterial pressure is >30 mmHg [2, 3]. Surgical pulmonary endarterectomy (PEA) is considered a permanently curative treatment option and is therefore recommended as the fist-line treatment [4, 5]. Having the potential to gradually remove mechanical obstruction of the pulmonary tree, the ultimate objective of BPA should be reducing mortality and improving quality of life (QoL) of patients with CTEPH. To date, a survival benefit of BPA has been hypothesized but not yet clearly demonstrated. No direct comparisons between PEA and BPA have been performed and BPA is considered a reasonable therapeutic option only once surgery has been excluded [5]. Further,

despite the fact that there is an area of overlap between diseases amenable to PEA and BPA, the two techniques basically address different anatomical patterns and setting a randomized comparison represents a difficult challenge. Attempts to generate indirect comparisons from available literature and historical CTEPH cohorts are encouraging but they are fraught with potential selection biases [6–8]. Remarkably, in a large French series of patients with not-operated CTEPH, BPA was independently associated with improved survival [9]. Indeed, excellent survival after BPA has been reported by numerous authors [10–13]. The RACE trial (ClinicalTrials.gov Identifier: NCT02634203) is a head-to-head comparison of BPA with riociguat, an oral stimulator of soluble guanylate cyclase and, to date, the only drug approved for inoperable CTEPH or persistent/recurrent PH after PEA. Results of the RACE trial will be relevant, although a) riociguat was not demonstrated to improve survival in

CTEPH patients; b) the primary endpoint is a surrogate endpoint, i.e., change from baseline in pulmonary vascular resistance (PVR); and c) the role of BPA could be seen in most instances as complementary rather than alternative to targeted medical treatment.

Functional class and exercise capacity. Important changes in New York Heart Association (NYHA) or the World Health Organization (WHO) functional class after BPA have been consistently reported. For example, in the French experience, patients with NYHA functional class III or IV were 64.7% at baseline and 21.3% after the last BPA [12]. In another study, the corresponding figures were 96% at baseline and 20.8% after the last BPA [14]. The UK registry reported a decrease in the rate of patients with WHO functional class ≥ 3 from 80% to 13% (p < 0.0001) [15].

Similarly, several studies demonstrated a progressive improvement in exercise capacity after BPA. In the largest Japanese experience, the 6-min walk distance (6MWD) increased from 318 ± 122 m at baseline to 401 ± 105 at the end of BPA, with a further increase to 430 ± 109 during follow-up [16]. Another Japanese series reported a mean 6MWD increase of 106 m [8]. In Europe, an average increase in 6MWD of 33 meters was reported in the German experience [17], 45 m in the French registry [12], 74 m in the UK [15], 54 m in a Czech series [14].

Of interest, previous surgical studies demonstrated an independent association between postoperative 6MWD and 1-year survival [18].

Quality of life. Improved quality of life (QoL) after BPA has been consistently reported using different parameters such as EQ-5D questionnaire [14] and the Cambridge Pulmonary Hypertension Outcome Review (CAMPHOR) [15].

10.3   Surrogate Efficacy Endpoints

Hemodynamics. Consistent reductions of mean pulmonary artery pressure (mPAP) and PVR after BPA have been observed in all Japanese series, and these results were confirmed during long-term follow-up [8, 16]. In Europe, the German registry [17] reported an 18% decline in

mPAP and a 26% decline in PVR after BPA. Similarly, in the France registry a reduction in mPAP by 30% and in PVR by 49% was achieved [12].

Mean PAP >30 mmHg is significantly associated with worst clinical outcomes in medically treated patients with CTEPH [3]. After PEA, mPAP of ≥ 38 mm Hg correlated with worse long-term survival [19] and postoperative PVR was found to be an independent risk factor for in-hospital and 1-year mortality [18, 19]. The principal goal of BPA should be the relief of PH so the same target of PEA seems reasonable: reduction of mPAP below 25 mmHg [13, 20, 21]. Nevertheless, even with PEA this target is achievable in <50% of the patients, and the <30 mm Hg mean PAP threshold could be a reasonable alternative in many patients. Indeed, this threshold was associated with good clinical outcomes in medically treated patients [3] and after PEA [19], and it is used by many experienced centers as the BPA target [8]. Of note, the benefits of BPA on hemodynamics cannot be estimated immediately at the time of the procedure, as significant changes were observed in a large proportion of patients only around 6 months after the procedure [1, 22].

On the other hand, some patients experience shortness of breath during exercise despite normalization of rest mPAP. Exercise PH is thought to be the principal mechanism of reduced exercise capacity in these patients [23], advocating for a more aggressive approach especially in younger patients.

Right ventricular function. Right-heart failure is the main cause of death in patients with PH, and its prognostic role is certainly superior to the role of PVR [24]. Through the progressive right ventricle (RV) unloading, BPA has been associated with improved RV function and reverse RV remodeling [17, 25–27]. Indeed, significant ameliorations have been described in all measures of RV function, including volume, ejection fraction, tricuspid annular plane systolic excursion (TAPSE), and RV free wall peak strain.

Arterial oxygen saturation and need for home oxygen therapy. A number of studies have demonstrated increase in arterial oxygen saturation after BPA [10, 15, 22, 28]. The beneficial impact of BPA on arterial saturation allows patients to withdraw from oxygen therapy. Hence, oxygen saturation > 95% without home oxygen therapy should be considered an additional treatment goal of BPA.

Discontinuation of PH-specific drugs. Significant reduction or discontinuation of medications for PH was reported in the first experience of refined BPA [10], and confirmed in subsequent studies even during long-term follow-up [8].

10.4 Safety Endpoints

Initial studies about BPA reported a high incidence of adverse events and fatal complications [29]. In recent years, after refinement of BPA techniques by Matsubara and colleagues [10], multiple reports demonstrated considerable improvement in procedural safety. In experienced hands, perioperative mortality is 0–3.4% [16]. However, the incidence of other intra- and postoperative complications remains not trivial [8, 30], although with decreasing rates after the learning curve [12]. The list of potential complications includes vessel perforation or rupture, dissection, hemoptysis, lung edema and/or hemorrhage, pneumothorax, contrast nephropathy, and vascular complications at the access site. Lung injury can result from wire manipulation or balloon over-dilation [31], as well as from reperfusion injury (RPI) [30].

An attempt to classify the severity of BPA complications is reported in Table 10.2. In general, they could be classified as life-threatening (requiring intubation; mechanical ventilation; extracorporeal membrane oxygenation; bleedings 5, 3b, or 3c according to the Bleeding Academic Research Consortium, BARC [33]; retroperitoneal hematoma; cardiogenic shock); severe (requiring noninvasive positive pressure ventilation, bleeding BARC 3a, AKI 3, major access-site complications, unplanned surgical intervention, unplanned endovascular intervention associated with severe bleeding); moderate (requiring prolonged supplemental oxygenation, prolonged hospitalization, unplanned

Table 10.2 Clinical classification of adverse events of BPA

Classification	Parameter
Life-threatening	Requiring intubation Mechanical ventilation Extracorporeal membrane oxygenation Life-threatening bleedings (BARC 5, 3b, or 3c[a]) Retroperitoneal hematoma Cardiogenic shock
Severe	Requiring noninvasive positive pressure ventilation Acute kidney injury class 3 Severe bleeding (BARC 3a[a]) Major access-site complications (arteriovenous fistula, pseudoaneurysm, irreversible nerve injury) Unplanned surgical intervention Unplanned endovascular intervention associated with severe bleeding
Moderate	Requiring prolonged supplemental oxygenation Prolonged hospitalization Unplanned endovascular intervention without severe bleeding Acute kidney injury class 2
Mild	Managed conservatively Requiring only temporary supplemental oxygenation Acute kidney injury class 1

BARC Bleeding Academic Research Consortium.
[a]BARC 5 = fatal bleeding, BARC 3a = overt bleeding plus hemoglobin drop of 3 to <5 g/dL (provided that hemoglobin drop is related to bleed); transfusion with overt bleeding; BARC 3b = overt bleeding plus hemoglobin drop <5 g/dL (provided that hemoglobin drop is related to bleed); cardiac tamponade; bleeding requiring surgical intervention for control; bleeding requiring IV vasoactive agents; BARC 3c = intracranial hemorrhage confirmed by autopsy, imaging, or lumbar puncture; intraocular bleed compromising vision [32].

endovascular intervention without severe bleeding, AKI class 2); or mild (managed conservatively, requiring only temporary supplemental oxygenation and/or manageable with endovascular treatment). It is still unclear if mild lung opacities on chest radiograph and/or CT scan without hypoxemia and without hemoptysis should be considered as procedural complications or if they are just a transient effect of reperfusion.

Results from different cohorts suggest that the rate of complication after BPA is closely related to the severity of PH and PVR at the time of BPA

[12, 34]. Historically, Inami and colleagues developed the Pulmonary Edema Predictive Scoring Index (PEPSI) to integrate the efficacy of the procedure, as measured by sum total change of pulmonary flow grade (*see definition below*), with the risk of developing reperfusion edema, which has a strong correlation with baseline PVR. Thus, PEPSI was defined as sum total change of pulmonary flow grade (PFG) during BPA x baseline PVR (wood units). A safety threshold of 35.4 was identified by ROC curve analysis, with a sensitivity of 88.7%, a specificity of 82.8%, positive predictive value of 75.8%, and negative predictive value of 92.3% [1]. Importantly, however, in almost all Japanese and experienced BPA centers, with refined modern BPA technique, a large number of lesions are often treated during the initial procedure. In most of these cases PEPSI would be very high, whereas rates of RPI are negligible. The predictive value of PEPSI with the modern BPA technique has been therefore questioned.

10.5 Lesion-Level Outcomes

Residual stenosis. There is general consensus about the difficulty in judging the success of BPA at the target lesion level through measurement of residual vessel diameter or area stenosis, as com-

monly evaluated for percutaneous coronary intervention (PCI). BPA acts, in fact, through mechanisms which are quite different from PCI on atherosclerotic lesions [35]. Even if a relationship between residual stenosis and efficacy of the procedure is likely, there is no validated threshold to use this parameter as an efficacy measure. In refined BPA, use of undersized balloons is initially recommended in order to reduce reperfusion injury and allow the vessel to gradually regain the original size before optimizing results with larger balloons, further complicating the use of residual diameter stenosis as a proxy for procedural success at the lesion level.

Pulmonary flow grade. Evaluation of flow in the pulmonary circulation is based on the observation of both antegrade flow distal to the target lesions and rate of contrast clearance from the bed of perfused pulmonary veins [1]. Classification of pulmonary perfusion as suggested by Inami and colleagues is reported in Table 10.3. The authors demonstrated that the sum total change of pulmonary flow grade (PFG) scores at the time of the BPA, differently from the total number of target vessels, was significantly correlated with the change in PVR and mean PAP at follow-up [1].

Ratio of pressures across the target lesion. The ratio of distal to proximal pressures across the target lesion (Pd/Pa) can be measured with

Table 10.3 Definition of pulmonary flow grade

Grading	Description
Grade 0	No perfusion or penetration with minimal perfusion of pulmonary arteries
Grade 1	Partial perfusion of pulmonary arteries *Visualization of the pulmonary artery bed distal to the lesion but the rate of entry of contrast material into the vessels distal to the lesion or its rate of clearance from the distal bed of pulmonary artery is perceptibly slower than its entry into or clearance from comparable areas not perfused by the target vessel*
Grade 2	Complete perfusion of pulmonary arteries and partial perfusion of pulmonary veins *Antegrade flow into the bed of pulmonary artery distal to the lesions occurs as promptly as antegrade flow into the bed proximal to the lesions. However, the rate of appearance of contrast material from the bed of pulmonary veins perfused by the target pulmonary artery or the rate of contrast clearance from the bed of perfused pulmonary veins is perceptibly slower than that from comparable areas not perfused by the target vessel.*
Grade 3	Complete perfusion of both pulmonary arteries and veins

[a] Modified from Inami et al. [1].

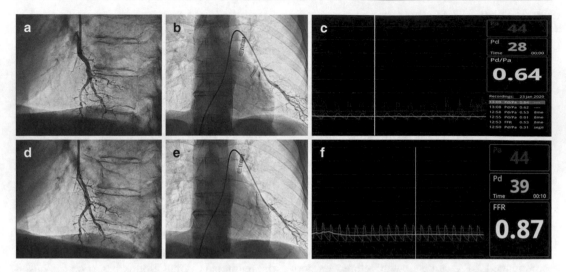

Fig. 10.1 Additional value of distal to proximal pressures ratio over pulmonary flow grade. (**a** and **b**) Angiography at anteroposterior (AP) and latero-lateral projection showing good angiographic result. PFG was classified as 3 also based on pulmonary vein flow. (**c**) Pd/Pa = 0.64. (**d** and **e**) Substantially unchanged angiographic appearance after additional balloon dilatation. (**f**) Final Pd/Pa = 0.87

coronary pressure wires and is an interesting and objective measure of efficacy of balloon dilatation at lesion level [1]. There is a strong correlation between the pulmonary flow grade score and the pressure ratios [36]. However, low Pd/Pa values were observed even in the presence of PFG 3, suggesting higher sensibility of pressure ratio in comparison with pulmonary flow (Fig. 10.1). An arbitrary Pd/Pa cutoff value >0.8 for an effective dilatation has been suggested, and its routine adoption could overcome the limitation of visual estimation of PFG and increase the effectiveness of balloon dilatations [36]. Measurement of distal pressure was also proposed to increase procedural safety. Indeed, following previous observations that the median value of mPAP before angioplasty in patients without lung reperfusion injury was 33 mm Hg, a threshold of 35 mm Hg distal mPAP is currently recommended in order to reduce the risk of reperfusion injury [1, 36].

10.6 Patient-Tailored Treatment Goal [21]

The ultimate objective of BPA is to cure PH [20] and improve survival. In parallel, BPA treatment is considered completely accomplished when patients are free of symptoms, home oxygen therapy, and PH-specific drugs. Nonetheless, a considerable number of patients undergoing BPA were excluded from PEA because of severe comorbidity or excessively high surgical risk. In this patient population, including many elderly patients, a different treatment goal can be established, taking into account safety and patient's subjective expectations. Hence, in some circumstances patient's satisfaction (patients believe that they no longer require additional BPA sessions) and improvement of QoL and exercise capacity can be considered as the principal objectives of BPA, along with cessation or reduction of specific PH drugs and oxygen therapy.

On the other end of the spectrum, there are young patients without severe comorbidity who are referred for BPA because of distal location of the disease deemed unfavorable for PEA. In these patients, normalization of mPAP at rest could be an insufficient target. Indeed residual stenoses could still be detected in many pulmonary arterial segments even after mPAP was normalized and it was reported that BPA can improve exercise capacity in some patients without PH at rest [20]. Residual stenoses generate ventilation-perfusion mismatch and dead-space ventilation, thus causing PH during exercise and effort dyspnea. A working hypothesis is that extensive revascularization by BPA (ERBPA) beyond hemodynamic normalization could provide clinical benefit. Indeed, in a small case series of CTEPH patients with normalized or borderline mPAP after BPA, ERBPA reduced the number of pulmonary arterial segments with residual stenoses from 11.7 ± 0.4 to 5.3 ± 0.5 segments, and improved symptoms, 6MWD, and VE/VCO2 slope in comparison with a control group of patients in the conventional BPA group [32].

10.7 Conclusions

The ultimate target of BPA should be relief of PH and improved survival. The best metric for success, to date, seems normalization of mPAP (<25 mmHg) as evaluated >6 months after the last procedure, in the absence of severe procedural complications. A number of additional clinical and surrogate endpoints at patient level can also be considered to evaluate procedural efficacy, although most of them lack useful thresholds to guide treatment. For some patients, because of advanced age or severe comorbidity, reasonable treatment goals can be reduction of symptoms, PH-specific drugs, and home oxygen therapy. In young and fit patients, optimization of BPA results with extensive revascularization beyond normalization of hemodynamics should be further investigated and could be encouraged, especially when effort dyspnea persists. At lesion level, treatment goals are normalization of pulmonary flow grade (PFR = 3) and reduction of ratio between distal and proximal pressure < 0.8.

References

1. Inami T, Kataoka M, Shimura N, Ishiguro H, Yanagisawa R, Taguchi H, Fukuda K, Yoshino H, Satoh T. Pulmonary edema predictive scoring index (PEPSI), a new index to predict risk of reperfusion pulmonary edema and improvement of hemodynamics in percutaneous transluminal pulmonary angioplasty. JACC Cardiovasc Interv. 2013;6:725–36.
2. Riedel M, Stanek V, Widimsky J, Prerovsky I. Longterm follow-up of patients with pulmonary thromboembolism. Late prognosis and evolu-

tion of hemodynamic and respiratory data. Chest. 1982;81:151–8.
3. Lewczuk J, Piszko P, Jagas J, Porada A, Wojciak S, Sobkowicz B, Wrabec K. Prognostic factors in medically treated patients with chronic pulmonary embolism. Chest. 2001;119:818–23.
4. Jamieson SW, Kapelanski DP, Sakakibara N, Manecke GR, Thistlethwaite PA, Kerr KM, Channick RN, Fedullo PF, Auger WR. Pulmonary endarterectomy: experience and lessons learned in 1,500 cases. Ann Thorac Surg. 2003;76:1457–62. discussion 1462-4
5. Konstantinides SV, Meyer G, Becattini C, Bueno H, Geersing GJ, Harjola VP, Huisman MV, Humbert M, Jennings CS, Jimenez D, Kucher N, Lang IM, Lankeit M, Lorusso R, Mazzolai L, Meneveau N, Ni Ainle F, Prandoni P, Pruszczyk P, Righini M, Torbicki A, Van Belle E, Zamorano JL. 2019 ESC guidelines for the diagnosis and management of acute pulmonary embolism developed in collaboration with the European Respiratory Society (ERS). Eur Heart J. 2020;41:543–603.
6. Zhang L, Bai Y, Yan P, He T, Liu B, Wu S, Qian Z, Li C, Cao Y, Zhang M. Balloon pulmonary angioplasty vs. pulmonary endarterectomy in patients with chronic thromboembolic pulmonary hypertension: a systematic review and meta-analysis. Heart Fail Rev. 2021;26:4.
7. Siennicka A, Darocha S, Banaszkiewicz M, Kedzierski P, Dobosiewicz A, Blaszczak P, Peregud-Pogorzelska M, Kasprzak JD, Tomaszewski M, Mroczek E, Zieba B, Karasek D, Ptaszynska-Kopczynska K, Mizia-Stec K, Mularek-Kubzdela T, Doboszynska A, Lewicka E, Ruchala M, Lewandowski M, Lukasik S, Chrzanowski L, Zielinski D, Torbicki A, Kurzyna M. Treatment of chronic thromboembolic pulmonary hypertension in a multidisciplinary team. Ther Adv Respir Dis. 2019;13:1753466619891529.
8. Aoki T, Sugimura K, Tatebe S, Miura M, Yamamoto S, Yaoita N, Suzuki H, Sato H, Kozu K, Konno R, Miyata S, Nochioka K, Satoh K, Shimokawa H. Comprehensive evaluation of the effectiveness and safety of balloon pulmonary angioplasty for inoperable chronic thrombo-embolic pulmonary hypertension: long-term effects and procedure-related complications. Eur Heart J. 2017;38:3152–9.
9. Taniguchi Y, Jais X, Jevnikar M, Boucly A, Weatherald J, Brenot P, Planche O, Parent F, Savale L, Fadel E, Montani D, Humbert M, Sitbon O, Simonneau G. Predictors of survival in patients with not-operated chronic thromboembolic pulmonary hypertension. J Heart Lung Transplant. 2019;38:833–42.
10. Mizoguchi H, Ogawa A, Munemasa M, Mikouchi H, Ito H, Matsubara H. Refined balloon pulmonary angioplasty for inoperable patients with chronic thromboembolic pulmonary hypertension. Circ Cardiovasc Interv. 2012;5:748–55.
11. Sugimura K, Fukumoto Y, Satoh K, Nochioka K, Miura Y, Aoki T, Tatebe S, Miyamichi-Yamamoto S,

Shimokawa H. Percutaneous transluminal pulmonary angioplasty markedly improves pulmonary hemodynamics and long-term prognosis in patients with chronic thromboembolic pulmonary hypertension. Circ J. 2012;76:485–8.

12. Brenot P, Jais X, Taniguchi Y, Garcia Alonso C, Gerardin B, Mussot S, Mercier O, Fabre D, Parent F, Jevnikar M, Montani D, Savale L, Sitbon O, Fadel E, Humbert M, Simonneau G. French experience of balloon pulmonary angioplasty for chronic thromboembolic pulmonary hypertension. Eur Respir J. 2019;53:5.

13. Inami T, Kataoka M, Yanagisawa R, Ishiguro H, Shimura N, Fukuda K, Yoshino H, Satoh T. Long-term outcomes after percutaneous transluminal pulmonary angioplasty for chronic thromboembolic pulmonary hypertension. Circulation. 2016;134:2030–2.

14. Jansa P, Heller S, Svoboda M, Pad'our M, Ambroz D, Dytrych V, Siranec M, Kovarnik T, Felsoci M, Hutyra M, Linhart A, Lindner J, Aschermann M. Balloon pulmonary angioplasty in patients with chronic thromboembolic pulmonary hypertension: impact on clinical and hemodynamic parameters, quality of life and risk profile. J Clin Med. 2020;9:1.

15. Hoole SP, Coghlan JG, Cannon JE, Taboada D, Toshner M, Sheares K, Fletcher AJ, Martinez G, Ruggiero A, Screaton N, Jenkins D, Pepke-Zaba J. Balloon pulmonary angioplasty for inoperable chronic thromboembolic pulmonary hypertension: the UK experience. Open Heart. 2020;7:e001144.

16. Ogawa A, Satoh T, Fukuda T, Sugimura K, Fukumoto Y, Emoto N, Yamada N, Yao A, Ando M, Ogino H, Tanabe N, Tsujino I, Hanaoka M, Minatoya K, Ito H II, Matsubara H. Balloon pulmonary angioplasty for chronic thromboembolic pulmonary hypertension: results of a multicenter registry. circ cardiovasc qual outcomes. Circulation. 2017;10:11.

17. Olsson KM, Wiedenroth CB, Kamp JC, Breithecker A, Fuge J, Krombach GA, Haas M, Hamm C, Kramm T, Guth S, Ghofrani HA, Hinrichs JB, Cebotari S, Meyer K, Hoeper MM, Mayer E, Liebetrau C, Meyer BC. Balloon pulmonary angioplasty for inoperable patients with chronic thromboembolic pulmonary hypertension: the initial German experience. Eur Respir J. 2017;49:5.

18. Mayer E, Jenkins D, Lindner J, D'Armini A, Kloek J, Meyns B, Ilkjaer LB, Klepetko W, Delcroix M, Lang I, Pepke-Zaba J, Simonneau G, Dartevelle P. Surgical management and outcome of patients with chronic thromboembolic pulmonary hypertension: results from an international prospective registry. J Thorac Cardiovasc Surg. 2011;141:702–10.

19. Cannon JE, Su L, Kiely DG, Page K, Toshner M, Swietlik E, Treacy C, Ponnaberanam A, Condliffe R, Sheares K, Taboada D, Dunning J, Tsui S, Ng C, Gopalan D, Screaton N, Elliot C, Gibbs S, Howard L, Corris P, Lordan J, Johnson M, Peacock A, MacKenzie-Ross R, Schreiber B, Coghlan G, Dimopoulos K, Wort SJ, Gaine S, Moledina S, Jenkins DP, Pepke-Zaba J. Dynamic risk stratification

of patient long-term outcome after pulmonary endarterectomy: results from the United Kingdom National Cohort. Circulation. 2016;133:1761–71.

20. Kataoka M, Inami T, Kawakami T, Fukuda K, Satoh T. Balloon pulmonary angioplasty (percutaneous transluminal pulmonary angioplasty) for chronic thromboembolic pulmonary hypertension: a Japanese perspective. JACC Cardiovasc Interv. 2019;12:1382–8.

21. Karyofyllis P, Demerouti E, Papadopoulou V, Voudris V, Matsubara H. Balloon pulmonary angioplasty as a treatment in chronic thromboembolic pulmonary hypertension: past, present, and future. Curr Treat Options Cardiovasc Med. 2020;22:7.

22. Kataoka M, Inami T, Hayashida K, Shimura N, Ishiguro H, Abe T, Tamura Y, Ando M, Fukuda K, Yoshino H, Satoh T. Percutaneous transluminal pulmonary angioplasty for the treatment of chronic thromboembolic pulmonary hypertension. Circ Cardiovasc Interv. 2012;5:756–62.

23. Kikuchi H, Goda A, Takeuchi K, Inami T, Kohno T, Sakata K, Soejima K, Satoh T. Exercise intolerance in chronic thromboembolic pulmonary hypertension after pulmonary angioplasty. Eur Respir J. 2020;56:1.

24. Van de Veerdonk MC, Kind T, Marcus JT, Mauritz GJ, Heymans MW, Bogaard HJ, Boonstra A, Marques KM, Westerhof N, Vonk-Noordegraaf A. Progressive right ventricular dysfunction in patients with pulmonary arterial hypertension responding to therapy. J Am Coll Cardiol. 2011;58:2511–9.

25. Broch K, Murbraech K, Ragnarsson A, Gude E, Andersen R, Fiane AE, Andreassen J, Aakhus S, Andreassen AK. Echocardiographic evidence of right ventricular functional improvement after balloon pulmonary angioplasty in chronic thromboembolic pulmonary hypertension. J Heart Lung Transplant. 2016;35:80–6.

26. Kimura M, Kohno T, Kawakami T, Kataoka M, Tsugu T, Akita K, Isobe S, Itabashi Y, Maekawa Y, Murata M, Fukuda K. Midterm effect of balloon pulmonary angioplasty on hemodynamics and subclinical myocardial damage in chronic thromboembolic pulmonary hypertension. Can J Cardiol. 2017;33:463–70.

27. Fukui S, Ogo T, Morita Y, Tsuji A, Tateishi E, Ozaki K, Sanda Y, Fukuda T, Yasuda S, Ogawa H, Nakanishi N. Right ventricular reverse remodelling after balloon pulmonary angioplasty. Eur Respir J. 2014;43:1394–402.

28. Roik M, Wretowski D, Labyk A, Kostrubiec M, Irzyk K, Dzikowska-Diduch O, Lichodziejewska B, Ciurzynski M, Kurnicka K, Golebiowski M, Pruszczyk P. Refined balloon pulmonary angioplasty driven by combined assessment of intra-arterial anatomy and physiology--multimodal approach to treated lesions in patients with non-operable distal chronic thromboembolic pulmonary hypertension--Technique, safety and efficacy of 50 consecutive angioplasties. Int J Cardiol. 2016;203:228–35.

29. Feinstein JA, Goldhaber SZ, Lock JE, Ferndandes SM, Landzberg MJ. Balloon pulmonary angioplasty

for treatment of chronic thromboembolic pulmonary hypertension. Circulation. 2001;103:10–3.

30. Hosokawa K, Abe K, Oi K, Mukai Y, Hirooka Y, Sunagawa K. Balloon pulmonary angioplasty-related complications and therapeutic strategy in patients with chronic thromboembolic pulmonary hypertension. Int J Cardiol. 2015;197:224–6.

31. Delcroix M, Torbicki A, Gopalan D, Sitbon O, Klok FA, Lang I, Jenkins D, Kim NH, Humbert M, Jais X, Noordegraaf AV, Pepke-Zaba J, Brenot P, Dorfmuller P, Fadel E, Ghofrani HA, Hoeper MM, Jansa P, Madani M, Matsubara H, Ogo T, Grunig E, D'Armini A, Galie N, Meyer B, Corkery P, Meszaros G, Mayer E, Simonneau G. ERS statement on chronic thromboembolic pulmonary hypertension. Eur Respir J. 2020;57:6.

32. Shinkura Y, Nakayama K, Yanaka K, Kinutani H, Tamada N, Tsuboi Y, Satomi-Kobayashi S, Otake H, Shinke T, Emoto N, Hirata KI. Extensive revascularisation by balloon pulmonary angioplasty for chronic thromboembolic pulmonary hypertension beyond haemodynamic normalisation. EuroIntervention. 2018;13:2060–8.

33. Mehran R, Rao SV, Bhatt DL, Gibson CM, Caixeta A, Eikelboom J, Kaul S, Wiviott SD, Menon V, Nikolsky E, Serebruany V, Valgimigli M, Vranckx P, Taggart D, Sabik JF, Cutlip DE, Krucoff MW, Ohman EM, Steg PG, White H. Standardized bleeding definitions for cardiovascular clinical trials: a consensus report from the bleeding academic research consortium. Circulation. 2011;123:2736–47.

34. Inami T, Kataoka M, Shimura N, Ishiguro H, Yanagisawa R, Kawakami T, Fukuda K, Yoshino H, Satoh T. Incidence, avoidance, and management of pulmonary artery injuries in percutaneous transluminal pulmonary angioplasty. Int J Cardiol. 2015;201:35–7.

35. Magon W, Stepniewski J, Waligora M, Jonas K, Przybylski R, Sikorska M, Podolec P, Kopec G. Virtual histology to evaluate mechanisms of pulmonary artery lumen enlargement in response to balloon pulmonary angioplasty in chronic thromboembolic pulmonary hypertension. J Clin Med. 2020;9:1.

36. Inami T, Kataoka M, Shimura N, Ishiguro H, Yanagisawa R, Fukuda K, Yoshino H, Satoh T. Pressure-wire-guided percutaneous transluminal pulmonary angioplasty: a breakthrough in catheter-interventional therapy for chronic thromboembolic pulmonary hypertension. JACC Cardiovasc Interv. 2014;7:1297–306.

Management of Complications During Balloon Pulmonary Angioplasty in Chronic Thromboembolic Pulmonary Hypertension

11

Ehtisham Mahmud and Lawrence Ang

11.1 Introduction

Balloon pulmonary angioplasty (BPA) was introduced over three decades ago as a potential treatment for inoperable chronic thromboembolic pulmonary hypertension (CTEPH) [1, 2], but remained poorly adopted due to the frequency of major complications. Since 2012, the techniques and equipment utilized for BPA have undergone multiple refinements with favorable outcomes and safety as reported from CTEPH centers worldwide. Here we review the historical and contemporary complications of BPA, and their clinical management.

11.2 Historical BPA Complications

The earliest described balloon angioplasty for pulmonary hypertension caused by pulmonary embolism was performed in 1986, wherein an 8 mm diameter balloon was used to dilate a band-like stenosis of the left basal lateral pulmonary artery segment [1]. After angioplasty the patient complained of a productive cough, and a chest X-ray image 24 h after the procedure showed pulmonary edema in the left latero-basal segment. At 36 h after the procedure the patient reported a persistent cough associated with expectoration of small amounts of hemorrhagic sputum and left lower lobe rales. This complication was ultimately considered to be due to reperfusion pulmonary edema (RPE) similar to that reported to occur after surgical thromboendarterectomy.

The earliest case series of 18 CTEPH patients treated with 47 BPA sessions in 2001 described the use of a soft-tipped 0.035 inch guidewire to traverse distally stenosed and occluded pulmonary arteries [2]. Initial dilation of stenoses was performed using 3–6 mm balloons. Intraprocedural complications occurred in four procedures, including one right lower lobe artery perforation from a stiff wire (2% of procedures) and three femoral artery pseudoaneurysms. RPE, defined as radiographic opacity in the dilated segment and worsening hypoxemia, developed in 11 of 18 patients (61% of patients; four occurring during BPA and seven occurring within 48 h after BPA). Three patients with RPE required mechanical ventilation (17% of total patients). One patient developed pulmonary edema in all dilated areas and died of right ventricular failure seven days after BPA (6% of total patients). Lessons drawn from these observed outcomes included the superior safety and efficacy of flexible wires over stiff wires, dispensability of systemic arterial cannulation, and frequency of RPE suggesting that BPA should be staged over multiple separate procedures.

E. Mahmud (✉) · L. Ang
Division of Cardiovascular Medicine, University of California, San Diego, CA, USA
e-mail: emahmud@ucsd.edu

11.3 BPA Evolution and Contemporary BPA Complications

A resurgence of BPA for CTEPH occurred in 2012 with multiple studies published from Japan [3–5]. In these reports, studying a range of 12–68 subjects per report, operators shared their observations when incorporating smaller diameter 1.5 and 2 mm balloons, thinner 0.014 inch guidewires, and intravascular imaging guidance into the BPA treatment regimen. Reported complication rates, including RPE (60–68%), hemoptysis (50%), wire perforation (3%), positive pressure ventilation (7%), mechanical ventilation (3–6%), percutaneous cardiopulmonary support (3%), and 12-month death (0–3%), revealed areas of interval improvement compared to earlier experiences.

Following these initial pioneering efforts, other reported BPA experiences worldwide have continued the use of smaller caliber 0.014 inch guidewires and balloon diameters as small as 2 mm [6–8]. From Norway (N = 20), reported complications included 7 instances of RPE (10% of procedures) and 2 deaths (10% of patients; one from acute right ventricular failure, one from acute pulmonary embolism). From Germany (N = 56, 266 procedures), 25 procedure-related complications occurred (32% of patients, 9.4% of procedures). The majority of these procedural complications were due to pulmonary vascular injury, including arterial dissection without bleeding (0.8%), arterial bleeding without hemoptysis (1.1%), and hemoptysis (5.6%). The reported incidence of RPE was low (0.8%). The most recent analysis from the University of California San Diego BPA Registry (N = 95; 402 procedures) reported asymptomatic lung vascular injury and uncomplicated hemoptysis in 1.5% and 8% of procedures, respectively [8]. The incidence of RPE, mechanical ventilation, or death was 0%.

Contemporary experience from the largest reported BPA cohort to date (N = 308; 1408 procedures), combining patients from multiple BPA centers across Japan, reflected improved procedural incidences of overall procedural complica-

tion (36.3%), including hemoptysis (14.0%), angiographic pulmonary artery perforation (2.9%), dissection (0.4%), and rupture (0.1%), compared to the initial Japanese results from 2012 [9]. Severe complications, including mechanical ventilation (5.5%), ECMO (2.9%), coil embolization (1.6%), and covered stenting (1.0%), were infrequently observed in this patient cohort. Twelve-month mortality after initial BPA therapy was 3.2%. Of note, the occurrence of reperfusion pulmonary edema initially reported through 2012 was replaced in these contemporary studies by more specific complication types as these are now considered to be a consequence of procedure-related pulmonary vascular injury. Lung injury in more contemporary studies is reported following the observance of post-BPA localized pulmonary infiltrates on chest X-ray or computer tomography (CT) imaging. The occurrence of BPA-related vascular injury by angiographic contrast extravasation was also identified as a major cause of lung injury identified by CT imaging [10], which historically may have been categorized as RPE.

11.4 Management of Complications During BPA

The most common complication occurring during BPA procedures is injury of the pulmonary artery (9.4% to 17.8%) sometimes leading to hemoptysis (5.6% to 14.0%) or associated with overt pulmonary artery dissection (0.4%) and rupture (0.1%). Known etiologies for pulmonary artery injury include distal wire perforation, balloon over-dilation, and high-pressure contrast injection [10]. Other rare intraprocedural complications include access-site vascular injury, acute kidney injury, or severe adverse reactions to contrast medium, moderate sedation, and local anesthesia. Management of pulmonary artery injury has three major aims: [1] treating vascular injury, [2] supporting respiratory function, and [3] avoiding cardiopulmonary failure.

Treating Vascular Injury Pulmonary artery injury, typically observed within the constellation of patient coughing, hemoptysis, and contrast extravasation by angiography, is generally considered to be associated with iatrogenic bleeding into the lung parenchyma (Fig. 11.1). This is initially managed by immediate balloon tamponade of the injured vessel (Table 11.1) as well as identification of the cause of injury. During instances of distal wire perforation, the wire is carefully repositioned back into a safe position. When balloon over-dilation occurs, care is taken not to reinjure the vessel during balloon tamponade, such as by using low-pressure inflation and optimizing the balloon position within a more suitable vessel segment. Cessation of additional systemic anticoagulation during initial management is prudent. For persistent bleeding despite initial treatments, repeat prolonged balloon tamponade [4, 8] and reversal of systemic anticoagulation may be employed (Fig. 11.2). It is for this reason that unfractionated heparin is routinely used for systemic anticoagulation and a low activated clotting time range of 200–250 s is targeted during BPA procedures. Reversal of heparin effects is typically achieved by administration of

intravenous protamine sulfate, dosed as 1 mg per 100 units of heparin used (maximum recommended dose of 50 mg), and slowly infused at a rate no greater than 5 mg per minute [11]. For partial reversal of anticoagulation, multiple lower doses of protamine can be administered in a stepwise fashion as needed. In severe cases of persistent pulmonary hemorrhage, bailout treatments using transcatheter coil embolization [2, 5, 12, 13], covered stent implantation [9, 10], and/or injection of gelatin or adipose into the target vessel have been previously described. In extreme circumstances, emergent surgery with chest tube insertion, hematoma evacuation, and/or lobectomy may be necessary to definitively manage bleeding (Fig. 11.3).

Supporting Respiratory Function Sentinel signs of pulmonary artery injury during BPA are the acute onset of patient coughing, hemoptysis, and contrast extravasation on angiography. When these signs occur, expectant management and a stepwise approach to maintain adequate

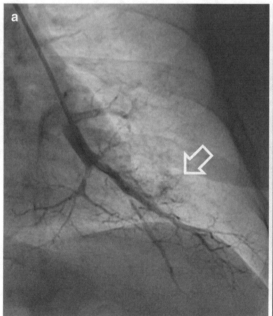
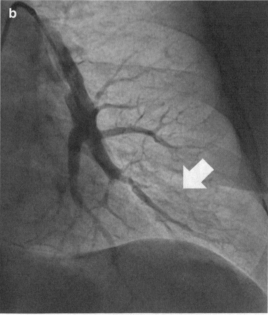

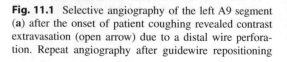

Fig. 11.1 Selective angiography of the left A9 segment (**a**) after the onset of patient coughing revealed contrast extravasation (open arrow) due to a distal wire perforation. Repeat angiography after guidewire repositioning and reversal of systemic anticoagulation without additional balloon tamponade (**b**) showed cessation of contrast extravasation (closed arrow)

respiratory function are prudent. Initial supplemental oxygenation by nasal cannula is helpful while simultaneously monitoring for bloody sputum. Patients who demonstrate preferential mouth breathing during this time may also be supported by face mask oxygenation and oropharyngeal suctioning. For suboptimal blood oxygenation despite these initial measures, administration of elevated concentrations of oxygen by face mask or high-flow nasal cannula may be warranted. Patients who demonstrate a greater degree of vascular injury and lung sequelae may

Table 11.1 Management of pulmonary artery perforation/rupture during BPA

1. Immediate balloon tamponade of the injured pulmonary artery
2. Oxygenation support including oropharyngeal suctioning, supplemental oxygen, noninvasive positive pressure ventilation (mechanical ventilation and ECMO in respiratory failure)
3. Cessation/reversal of anticoagulation
4. Repeat prolonged balloon tamponade as necessary
5. For persistent pulmonary hemorrhage consider bailout transcatheter coil embolization, covered stent implantation, and/or gelatin/adipose injection

need to be supported with noninvasive positive airway pressure in addition to administration of high-concentration oxygen [3, 4]. The use of diuretic and inhaled nitric oxide therapy has been previously described for the treatment of reperfusion pulmonary edema [2, 6], but its utility for improving oxygenation due to pulmonary hemorrhage is not clearly established. Infrequently, patients with severe pulmonary vascular injury and respiratory complications during BPA need to be supported with endotracheal intubation and mechanical ventilation in order to maintain adequate respiratory function and facilitate the ongoing management of concurrent vascular and/or hemodynamic abnormalities.

Management of Cardiopulmonary Failure
Patients with CTEPH undergoing BPA treatment have baseline compromised pulmonary reserve due to ventilation-perfusion mismatch and frequent need for continuous supplemental oxygen therapy. These patients may also have compromised cardiac reserve due to long-standing pulmonary hypertension and right ventricular dysfunction. In the context of suffering severe

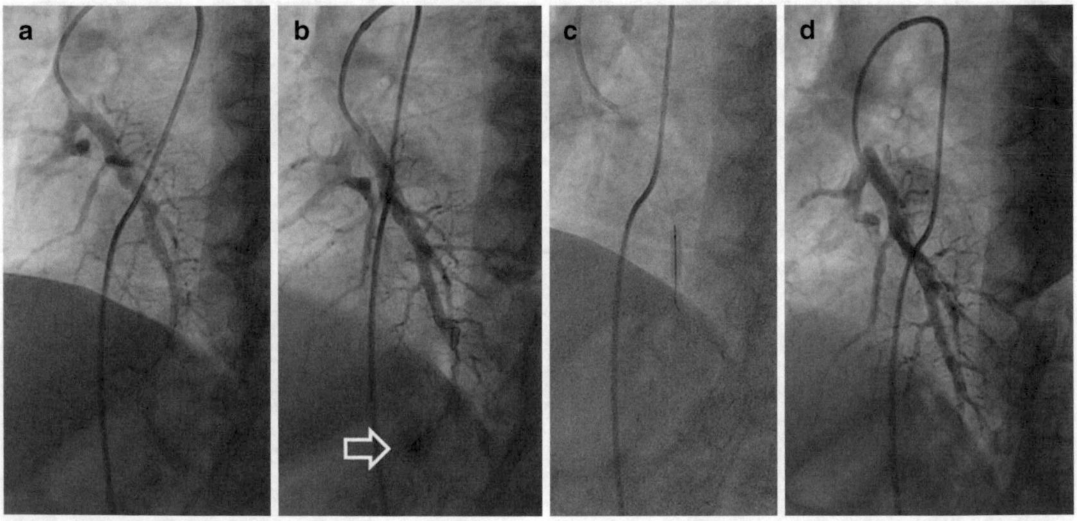

Fig. 11.2 A guidewire and 2 mm compliant balloon are positioned in the distal right lower lobe A10 branch (**a**). Patient coughing and hemoptysis ensued immediately after balloon angioplasty, followed by repeat angiography (**b**) showing distal vessel contrast extravasation (arrow). Treatment of pulmonary vascular injury included step-wise reversal of systemic anticoagulation, guidewire repositioning, and repeat prolonged balloon tamponade using a 3 mm compliant balloon (**c**). Final angiography showed cessation of contrast extravasation (**d**) and clinical hemostasis was achieved

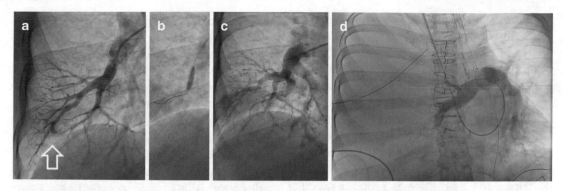

Fig. 11.3 Distal wire perforation of a right lower lobe branch (**a**) is observed as contrast extravasation on segmental pulmonary angiograms (arrow). Systematic anticoagulation was fully reversed, repeat prolonged balloon tamponade was performed (**b**), and angiographically apparent hemostasis was achieved (**c**). However, occult pulmonary hemorrhage during post-BPA observation led to a large right hemothorax, complicated by right lung collapse and marked mass effect on mediastinal structures (**d**), which was treated with endotracheal intubation, chest tube insertion, extracorporeal membrane oxygenation support, and surgery

pulmonary vascular injury and pulmonary hemorrhage during BPA, a patient's respiratory function may be further compromised leading to severe hypoxemia, further depression of cardiac function, and initiation of a vicious cycle of cardiopulmonary and multiorgan failure. This process may explain the link between significant pulmonary edema occurring after BPA treatment and patient mortality described within multiple BPA reports. Feinstein et al. [2] described one patient who developed segmental pulmonary edema in all dilated areas, was treated with mechanical ventilatory support and inhaled nitric oxide, suffered right ventricular failure, and died 1 week after BPA. Mizoguchi et al. [5] described one patient with severe reperfusion lung injury that led to worsening of right ventricular failure despite percutaneous cardiopulmonary support and eventual death. Conversely, they also observed that none of the patients with only mild lung injury, identified by chest CT imaging alone, required intratracheal intubation. Kataoka et al. [4] described one patient with severe post-BPA pulmonary edema that needed both mechanical ventilation and percutaneous cardiopulmonary support. Olsson et al. [7] described a fatal episode of pulmonary bleeding due to a right lower lobe artery wire perforation that ultimately led to a large right-sided hemothorax, respiratory distress, and shock that could

not be stabilized. Andreassen et al. [6] described the death of one patient that occurred 2 h after initial BPA therapy and was associated with both BPA-related pulmonary edema and postmortem verification of right ventricular failure. Finally, the two leading causes of post-BPA mortality from the multicenter Japanese registry [9] were severe right-heart failure related to CTEPH and multiorgan failure.

From these experiences, operators from different BPA centers have offered various strategies to avoid serious complications and death. Voorberg et al. [1] suggested that it may be advisable to dilate fewer segments in a single session because complications occurring in all treated segments could result in severe respiratory insufficiency. Feinstein et al. [2] suggested superior safety and efficacy using flexible rather than stiff guidewires during intervention, and that BPA should be performed in a staged fashion over multiple separate procedures. Furthermore, the potential for severe reperfusion pulmonary edema, especially in patients with baseline mean pulmonary artery pressure > 35 mmHg, should be anticipated prior to performing BPA. Mizoguchi et al. [5] supported the use of 0.014 inch guidewires and low-profile balloon catheters to lower the risk of vessel perforation, and treatment of fewer vessels during initial BPA sessions (such as fewer vessels within fewer lobes) to reduce the lung area at risk of reperfusion pulmonary edema. Similarly, Andreassen et al. [6] supported performing multiple shorter procedures with a limited number of dilations performed during each procedure. Sugimura et al. [3] attributed the occurrence of less severe complications to the user of smaller diameter balloons and treatment of fewer lobes per procedure. Mizoguchi et al. and Sugimura et al. also described the adjunctive use of intravascular ultrasound and optical coherence tomography imaging to optimize BPA treatment, respectively. Other suggested measures to decrease the risk of pulmonary artery perforation include proper wire positioning, knuckle-wire technique, and cautious approach to treating occluded pulmonary artery segments [14].

Despite the aforementioned strategies to optimize BPA technique and avoid serious complications, the management of severe pulmonary vascular injury should aim to sufficiently support both respiratory and circulatory function. Immediate control of bleeding as previously described should be achieved if possible. If first-line noninvasive positive pressure ventilation does not pneumatically suppress pulmonary hemorrhage or maintain adequate oxygenation, then mechanical intubation should be quickly performed [15]. In the context of significant bleeding into a unilateral airway and massive hemoptysis, lateral decubitus positioning towards the impaired lung and endobronchial intubation of the contralateral lung may be warranted. In the context of significant bleeding into the pleural space and occurrence of tension hemothorax, then emergent chest tube insertion, central line insertion, fluid resuscitation, and blood transfusion should be performed. Additional support with extracorporeal membrane oxygenation (ECMO) for ongoing respiratory and circulatory failure can be used to rescue and stabilize patients. In these extreme cases, ECMO may be useful as a bridge to emergency surgical and nonsurgical interventions for recalcitrant bleeding as well as cardiopulmonary recovery.

11.5 Conclusions

Contemporary BPA and management of complications are the products of continuous refinements of the techniques and equipment used to perform BPA, deeper understanding of the mechanisms of lung injury, and multifaceted approach to addressing complications. A methodical approach is currently used to terminate bleeding, support respiratory function, and avoid cardiopulmonary failure when complications occur. Global adoption of BPA, worldwide reporting of treatment successes and complications, and shared learning have contributed to both improved patient outcomes and lowered incidence of complications since its inception.

References

1. Voorburg JA, Cats VM, Buis B, Bruschke AV. Balloon angioplasty in the treatment of pulmonary hypertension caused by pulmonary embolism. Chest. 1988;94:1249–53.
2. Feinstein JA, Goldhaber SZ, Lock JE, Ferndandes SM, Landzberg MJ. Balloon pulmonary angioplasty for treatment of chronic thromboembolic pulmonary hypertension. Circulation. 2001;103:10–3.
3. Sugimura K, Fukumoto Y, Satoh K, et al. Percutaneous transluminal pulmonary angioplasty markedly improves pulmonary hemodynamics and long-term prognosis in patients with chronic thromboembolic pulmonary hypertension. Circ J. 2012;76:485–8.
4. Kataoka M, Inami T, Hayashida K, et al. Percutaneous transluminal pulmonary angioplasty for the treatment of chronic thromboembolic pulmonary hypertension. Circ Cardiovasc Interv. 2012;5:756–62.
5. Mizoguchi H, Ogawa A, Munemasa M, Mikouchi H, Ito H, Matsubara H. Refined balloon pulmonary angioplasty for inoperable patients with chronic thromboembolic pulmonary hypertension. Circ Cardiovasc Interv. 2012;5:748–55.
6. Andreassen AK, Ragnarsson A, Gude E, Geiran O, Andersen R. Balloon pulmonary angioplasty in patients with inoperable chronic thromboembolic pulmonary hypertension. Heart. 2013;99:1415–20.
7. Olsson KM, Wiedenroth CB, Kamp JC, et al. Balloon pulmonary angioplasty for inoperable patients with chronic thromboembolic pulmonary hypertension: the initial German experience. Eur Respir J. 2017;49:1602409.
8. Mahmud E, Patel M, Ang L, Poch D. Advances in balloon pulmonary angioplasty for chronic thromboembolic pulmonary hypertension. Pulm Circ. 2021;11:2.

9. Ogawa A, Satoh T, Fukuda T, Sugimura K, Fukumoto Y, Emoto N, Yamada N, Yao A, Ando M, Ogino H, Tanabe N, Tsujino I, Hanaoka M, Minatoya K, Ito J, Matsubara H. Balloon pulmonary angioplasty for chronic thromboembolic pulmonary hypertension: results of a multicenter registry. Circ Cardiovasc Qual Outcomes. 2017;10:e004029. https://doi.org/10.1161/CIRCOUTCOMES.117.004029.

10. Ejiri K, Ogawa A, Matsubara H. Bail-out technique for pulmonary artery rupture with a covered stent in balloon pulmonary angioplasty for chronic thromboembolic pulmonary hypertension. JACC Cardiovasc Interv. 2015;8:752–3.

11. "Protamine sulfate—drug summary." PDR.net. Prescriber's digital reference, 16 May, 2021

12. Baker CM, McGowan FX Jr, Keane JF, Lock JE. Pulmonary artery trauma due to balloon dilation:

recognition, avoidance, and management. J Am Coll Cardiol. 2000;36:1684–90.

13. Tajima H, Murata S, Kumazaki T, Abe Y, Takano T. Pulmonary artery perforation repair during thrombectomy using microcoil embolization. Cardiovasc Intervent Radiol. 2006;29:155–6.

14. Mahmud E, Madani MM, Kim NH, Poch D, Ang L, Behnamfar O, Patel MP, Auger WR. Chronic thromboembolic pulmonary hypertension: evolving therapeutic approaches for operative and inoperative disease. J Am Coll Cardiol. 2018;71:2468–86.

15. Hosokawa K, Abe K, Oi K, Mukai Y, Hirooka Y, Sunagawa K. Balloon pulmonary angioplasty-related complications and therapeutic strategy in patients with chronic thromboembolic pulmonary hypertension. Int J Cardil. 2015;197:224–6.

Balloon Pulmonary Angioplasty in Chronic Thromboembolic Pulmonary Hypertension: What Does the Future Hold?

Robert Zilinyi, Sanjum Sethi, and Ajay Kirtane

12.1 Introduction

In this chapter, we will discuss the future of balloon pulmonary angioplasty (BPA) in the algorithm of treatment modalities for the management of patients with chronic thromboembolic pulmonary hypertension (CTEPH). We will first briefly cover the advances in technique since the advent of the procedure, including more recent developments in adjunctive imaging modalities, utilization of advanced coronary techniques for chronic total occlusion lesions, and hybrid PEA-BPA techniques that have been reported. Given the rate at which BPA is being taken up across centers in Asia, North America, and Europe as a management technique for patients with CTEPH, we will discuss proposed evaluation and follow-up pathways as well as centers of excellence for patients with CTEPH as they are considered for pulmonary endarterectomy, BPA, medical management, or some combination thereof. We will then discuss ongoing questions that are being studied, including randomized controlled trials (RCTs) of BPA. And finally, we will discuss the lingering gaps in our knowledge, in particular the lack of long-term data on the efficacy and safety of BPA and the durability of its effects on pulmonary hemodynamics, functional class, and quality of life.

R. Zilinyi · S. Sethi · A. Kirtane (✉)
Columbia University Medical Center,
New York, NY, USA
e-mail: ak189@cumc.columbia.edu

12.2 Section 1: Current Techniques, Limitations, and Emerging Techniques

Brief History of Modern Technique: To understand where the field of BPA currently stands as regards modern technique, we will briefly discuss the history of BPA up until this point, focusing on the changes in technique over the years. As this content has been covered in detail in previous chapters, the following description is not meant to be exhaustive but rather used as a refresher. For complete details on history, evolution of technique, and clinical outcomes, please see Chaps. 5, 6, 7.

The first BPA series was reported by Feinstein et al. in 2001 describing 18 patients with CTEPH who underwent BPA [1]. The technique utilized by Feinstein et al. utilized high tip load wires, balloons sized up to 100% of the target vessel diameter with relatively few sessions per patient, and up to 4 lobes treated in a single session. Although significant improvements were observed in mean pulmonary arterial pressure (mPAP), 6-minute walk distance (6MWD), and NYHA class, due to a high rate of procedure-related complications, including a 5.5% mortality rate, the procedure was largely abandoned for several years. In 2012, Kataoko et al. and later Mizoguchi et al. described their refined techniques for BPA, opting for undersized balloons, or balloons sized with intravas-

© Springer Nature Switzerland AG 2022
F. Saia et al. (eds.), *Balloon pulmonary angioplasty in patients with CTEPH*,
https://doi.org/10.1007/978-3-030-95997-5_12

cular ultrasound (IVUS), and limiting sessions to single lobes of the lung with a limited number of lesions treated per session [2, 3]. These refined techniques saw similar improvements in pulmonary hemodynamics and quality-of-life markers (6MWD, NYHA/WHO FC) as did Feinstein et al. with lower mortality rates, albeit still with a high procedure-related complication rate (predominantly what was felt to be reperfusion pulmonary edema (RPE) at the time). Since that time, the Japanese groups have continued to refine their techniques, with Inami et al. describing the pulmonary edema predictive scoring index (PEPSI), aimed at decreasing the rate of BPA-related RPE or injury [4]. This technique utilizes pressure wire guidance to better characterize pulmonary flow grade and a scoring index which is the product of the baseline pulmonary vascular resistance (PVR) multiplied by the sum total of pulmonary flow grade change, to predict and reduce RPE and vessel injury.

Over the last 7 years, several European and American centers have started BPA programs and have reported their initial experiences [5–11]. There is significant heterogeneity in the reported techniques. However, the initial lessons learned from the experience of Feinstein et al. with oversized balloons and treatment of multiple lobes in a given session appear to have been heeded by most. The general modern technique, more fully detailed by Dr. Matsubara in Chap. 5, utilizes a long sheath/guide catheter system to gain appropriate access to the desired pulmonary artery and segmental vasculature. Once in the appropriate vessel with target lesion identified via selective pulmonary angiography, the desired lesion is crossed, generally with a low tip load 0.014″ guidewire closely followed by a small-diameter monorail balloon (often 2 mm x 20 mm) for initial dilation. The next steps, including the performance of subsequent dilations, the sizing of subsequent balloons, the number of dilations per session, and whether serial dilations of a given lesions will occur within the same or sequential sessions, vary by institution and operator. Most operators will limit their interventions to a single lung per session, if not a single lobe,

and opt for multiple sessions to progressively improve the pulmonary hemodynamics and functional class. Patients are generally monitored for 24–48 hours postoperatively for procedure-related complications, which have decreased over the years.

Advances in Imaging: Although several Japanese centers have been using IVUS to guide their BPA interventions since their first reports in 2012, other centers have demonstrated less enthusiasm for routine use of intravascular imaging in BPA. However, over the last several years, there has been an increase in reports of various intravascular and cross-sectional adjunctive imaging modalities being used in BPA [12–18]. Roik et al. have published a report detailing one of the most comprehensive experiences of combining adjunctive imaging modalities and real-time hemodynamic assessments to guide their BPA innterventions [16]. In 9 patients undergoing serial BPA, the authors utilized 3D rotational angiography, optical coherence tomography (OCT), IVUS, and PEPSI-PWG technique (proposed by Inami et al.) [4] to guide their BPA interventions, with a low reported procedure-related complication rate. The results of this study, although compelling, are limited by the small sample size and use of multiple adjunctive modalities, which make it difficult to ascertain where the potential benefit in reduction of adverse events is being derived from.

The remainder of the current literature exploring new adjunctive imaging modalities has predominantly been feasibility and safety studies to examine the potential role of such modalities as C-arm CT (CACT) and DynaCT post-processing software to deliver 3D angiographic reconstructions to be used in conjunction with traditional digital subtraction angiography (DSA) as a road map to better guide BPA interventions [12, 13, 15–17]. Maschke et al. reported their experience in 2019 with 266 BPA procedures in 67 patients utilizing a selective CACT 3D rendering of the pulmonary vasculature semi-transparently superimposed over real-time fluoroscopy images to guide their BPAs [13]. Lin et al. published a retrospective study in 2020 of 175 BPA procedures in 34 patients comparing DynaCT 3D reconstruction in addition to traditional DSA (23 patients) with DSA alone (11 patients) to guide BPA [15]. The 2D group underwent traditional BPA similar in technique to what is described above. The 3D group underwent contrast-enhanced selective DynaCT of the lobe with the target lesions. Through the use of post-processing software and a balloon that automatically tracks the angle position of the 3D image, the angle of the C-arm is automatically adjusted to optimize the angle of view of the desired vessel, after which super-selective angiography is performed of the target vessel and BPA is performed in the same manner as was performed in the 2D group. Some of the most compelling details of this report are the decrease in radiation exposure for both patient and operator (DAP/hr. 1346.83 µGy m [2]/hr. vs. 2561.76 µG m [2]/hr., p < 0.001 for 3D and 2D, respectively) and increase in the number of total lesions treated per session (5.83 vs. 3.73, p = 0.008 for 3D and 2D, respectively) in a shorter period of time per session (3.58 hr. vs. 4.49 hr., p = 0.002 for 3D and 2D, respectively) with lower total contrast used (225.22 mL vs. 292.73 mL, p = 0.013 for 3D and 2D, respectively).

The primary procedure-related complication of BPA was previously felt to be RPE akin to what is observed in patients post-PEA. All of the early literature cites RPE as the primary complication of BPA, given the post-procedural appearance of new opacities in the lobes which were recently reperfused on standard chest radiographs or CT imaging, associated with hypoxia and occasionally hemoptysis. Recently, several groups have suggested that perhaps RPE does not exist in BPA in the same way that it does in PEA, and that what was previously felt to be RPE actually represents pulmonary parenchymal hemorrhage due to distal wire perforation, balloon overdilation, or high-pressure contrast injection [19, 20]. If further studies continue to support this more recent hypothesis, and most procedure-related complications are in fact iatrogenic, further advances in imaging and BPA techniques may hold serious promise for the future of BPA.

Difficult-to-treat lesions: Early experiences with BPA, including Feinstein et al., Mizoguchi

et al., and Kataoka et al., generally chose to treat all targetable lesions as equal. Given the paucity of experience with BPA at the time, there was no formal classification of BPA lesions or knowledge that lesions might behave differently in success and complication rates [1–3]. In 2016, Kawakami et al. described a novel angiographic classification of BPA lesions (Fig. 12.1), which has subsequently been adopted by many as the standard classification of CTEPH lesions for BPA in the literature [21]. In their report, although the vast majority of CTEPH lesions fall under types A–C, the highest rate of procedure-related complications occurred in type E lesions (tortuous), followed by type C lesions (subtotal occlusions) and type D lesions (CTO lesions). The higher rate of complications in type C lesions compared with type D lesions was felt to be attributable to the higher failure rate of CTO BPA interventions in that cohort (13.5% for type C lesions vs. 47.8% in type D lesions), but that otherwise, type D lesions were higher risk if able to be treated. These findings of higher rates of complications with type D and E lesions have led some operators to eliminate treatment of these lesions altogether from their practice. Kurzyna et al. in 2017 described their shift from treatment of all possible BPA lesions (including type D and E lesions) to treating only ring and web lesions (type A and B lesions), comparing the outcomes between their initial experience and the subsequent change in their approach [22]. They observed a decrease in their procedure-related complications between the two groups, including cough, hemoptysis (mild, no difference in severe), vessel injury, and reperfusion lung injury of grade 3, 4, or 5 on the Inami classification [4, 5]. Most importantly, they observed a significant decrease in their procedure-related mortality (3 in initial cohort, 0 in the refined technique cohort).

Ikeda et al. in their 2019 paper evaluating independent predictors of procedure-related complications in BPA have further supported this finding, albeit with a slightly different classification scheme which did not include tortuous lesions [20]. They found that the only independent predictor of procedure-related complication

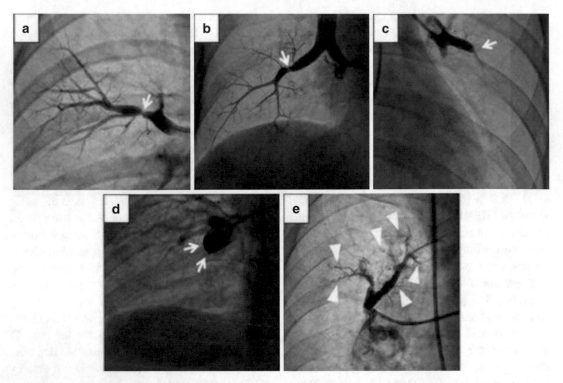

Fig. 12.1 Angiographic classification of the five types of chronic thromboembolic pulmonary hypertension lesions. The images included in this figure were taken from the original manuscript by Kawakami et al. in 2016. Panel (**a**) depicts a ring-type lesion. Panel (**b**) depicts a web lesion. Panel (**c**) depicts a subtotal lesion. Panel (**d**) depicts a total occlusion lesion. Panel (**e**) depicts a tortuous lesion. Kawakami T, Ogawa A, et al. Novel angiographic classification of each vascular lesion in chronic thromboembolic pulmonary hypertension based on selective angiogram and results of balloon pulmonary angioplasty. Circ Cardiovasc Interv. 2016; 9 (10):e003318

was treatment of occlusive type lesions (type D in Kawakami classification), highlighting the persistent difficulty of treating these lesions. While some have abandoned the treatment of these lesions, their persistence continues to present a problem for the patients with CTEPH undergoing BPA as these lesions represent areas of lung with little or no perfusion. Although not true of every center in which BPA is being practiced, many centers may avoid CTO and tortuous lesions. On the other hand, few groups are able to achieve resolution of pulmonary hypertension (PH), as defined by mPAP <25 mmHg, and in these series the operators tend to treat all available lesions until this endpoint is achieved [3, 4, 21, 23]. Without long-term outcome data available to us at this point, it is difficult to say whether there is a clinical benefit from achieving the goal of mPAP <25 mmHg, or if mPAP <30 mmHg is

sufficient. If, however, it appears that there is benefit to achieving this end, then a safe and reproducible treatment for CTO lesions might need to be pursued.

There have been reports in the literature regarding advanced techniques for safely approaching CTO lesions. Kawakami et al. in 2016 published their experience of utilizing a retrograde coronary CTO technique to treat a CTO CTEPH lesion in a 61-year-old man [24]. Most notable was the reduction in mPAP from baseline to post-BPA in the one CTO lesion (35 mmHg pre-BPA vs. 28 mmHg post-BPA). Nagayoshi et al. in 2017 subsequently described an IVUS-guided BPA of a CTO CTEPH lesion [14]. The authors report that they have performed this procedure on 5 total CTO lesions with 80% success rate and no significant procedure-related complications. Although the literature is sparse at this point, the development and implementation of a safe and reproducible approach for the treatment of CTO CTEPH lesions for BPA remain an important goal.

Hybrid procedures: The literature regarding hybrid techniques (BPA as an adjunct to PEA) is slightly more robust than that for effective treatment of CTO CTEPH lesions, although still limited. For patients with mixed lesions (predominantly proximal in one lung and distal in the other), for those with prohibitive preoperative hemodynamics for PEA, or in patients with either residual or recurrent PH following PEA, hybrid therapy with BPA appears to be a feasible option. Several authors have reported utilization of BPA preoperatively prior to PEA for a patient with pulmonary hemodynamics that made PEA surgery prohibitively high risk [25], concurrent with PEA surgery for patients with surgically inaccessible lesions on one side [26], and in a much larger and more heterogeneous cohort of patients with residual or recurrent PH post-PEA [2, 3, 27–29]. The time from PEA to BPA varies widely in this latter cohort, ranging from 7.3 months to 4.1 years [27–29]. As such, whether this group should be considered a hybrid therapy, rather than a salvage therapy for failure of the gold standard intervention due to multilevel disease or operator experience, is up for debate.

12.3 Section 2: Standardization of Evaluation, Follow-Up, and Reporting of Outcomes in Patients Undergoing BPA and the Need for Centers of Excellence in BPA

The field of BPA is rapidly expanding with new programs emerging across the United States, Europe, and Asia every year. As the field expands and operators continue to define and refine the optimal technique to maximize clinical benefit and minimize adverse events and complications, it is imperative that we standardize other aspects of BPA including pre-procedural assessment, follow-up, and reporting of outcomes and com-

plications to ensure uniformity and generalizability of results across the field. As the field of BPA is still in its infancy and lacks prospective randomized data comparing BPA with other recognized treatment modalities for CTEPH, it carries a class IIb recommendation from the European Society of Cardiology (ESC) for patients with inoperable CTEPH or those with an unfavorable risk/benefit ratio, below medical therapy with the guanylate cyclase activator, riociguat, which carries a class I recommendation in all patients with CTEPH with either residual or recurrent PH post-PEA or with surgically inaccessible disease [30]. This recommendation, albeit without formal society guidelines, has been upgraded by Kim et al. in the Proceedings of the sixth World Symposium on Pulmonary Hypertension section on CTEPH, where the authors suggest that BPA should be considered alongside initiation of medical therapy in patients who either fail PEA or are deemed nonoperative candidates [19].

There is no consensus or formal society guidelines for the appropriate workup of patients undergoing BPA, their routine follow-up, classification of procedure-related complications, or standardized reporting of patient outcomes and complications. Therefore, what follows hereafter represents a proposed standardized evaluation and follow-up algorithm, as well as proposed minimum standards for reporting of patient outcomes and complications. These views are exclusively those of the authors of this chapter and are meant as a starting point for discussion as parts of possible future guidelines or consensus statements.

Workup and follow-up: All patients with suspected CTEPH should undergo the standard diagnostic workup as outlined in Chap. 2 by Dr. Palazzini et al. The diagnostic algorithm for CTEPH recommended by the ESC is included in Fig. 12.2 for reference. This diagnostic algorithm has not changed in several years, although Kim et al. describe several recent advances in imaging including 3D dynamic lung perfusion MRI and cone beam CT (CBCT) which may one day supplant V/Q scans and DSA, respectively, on the diagnostic algorithm [19]. What remains undefined is the standard pre-BPA workup that all

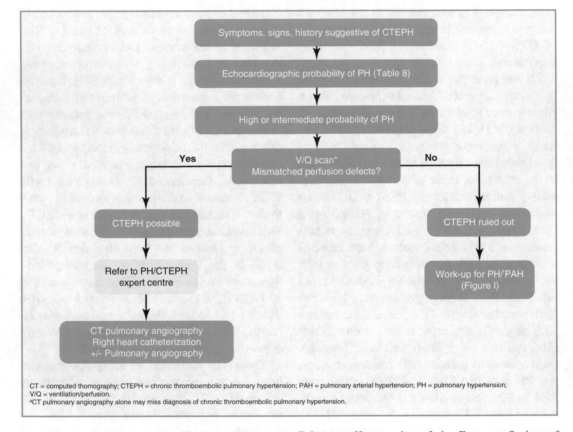

Fig. 12.2 Diagnostic algorithm for the diagnosis of chronic thromboembolic pulmonary hypertension according to the ESC/ERS 2015 guidelines for the diagnosis and management of pulmonary hypertension. Galiè N, Humbert M, et al. 2015 ESC/ERS Guidelines for the Diagnosis and Treatment of Pulmonary Hypertension: The Joint Taskforce for the Diagnosis and Treatment of Pulmonary Hypertension of the European Society of Cardiology (ESC) and the European Respiratory Society (ERS): Endorsed by: Association for European Paediatric and Congenital Cardiology (AEPC), International Society for Heart and Lung Transplantation (ISHLT). Eur Respir J. 2015; 46 (4):903–75

patients should undergo as well as the standard follow-up and intervals to such follow-up during BPA.

Figure 12.3 depicts our proposed algorithm for pre-BPA workup and follow-up during and after BPA. In addition to the standard tests and examinations involved in the diagnostic workup of a patient with CTEPH, including TTE, V/Q scan, CTPA, RHC, and DSA, we suggest that all patients undergo 6-minute walk test (6MWT), assessment of functional class (either NYHA or WHO classification), and serum levels of N-terminus pro-brain-type natriuretic peptide (NT-pro-BNP) prior to initiation of BPA. Performance on the 6MWT has long been used as the primary endpoint in studies examin-

ing PAH-targeted therapies, and was the primary endpoint in both the CHEST-1 and CHEST-2 trials for riociguat in CTEPH, which ultimately led to its FDA approval [31, 32]. Poor performance on the 6MWT has previously been associated with worse prognosis in patients with PAH [33]. Progressive PH and right-heart failure are ultimately the causes of death for most patients with CTEPH, and therefore patients should undergo routine evaluation for improvement or resolution of their PH throughout the course of their BPA sessions. Whether or not assessment and reporting of 6MWT and functional class should occur throughout the course of BPA treatment or simply after completion of all BPA treatment has not been clearly estab-

Fig. 12.3 Algorithm for standardized testing prior to, during, and after completion of balloon pulmonary angioplasty for the treatment of chronic thromboembolic pulmonary hypertension

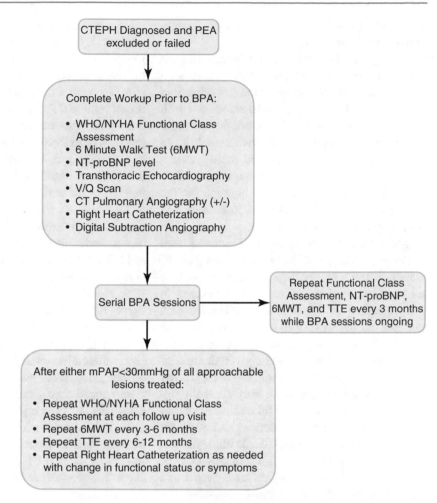

CTEPH Diagnosed and PEA excluded or failed

Complete Workup Prior to BPA:

- WHO/NYHA Functional Class Assessment
- 6 Minute Walk Test (6MWT)
- NT-proBNP level
- Transthoracic Echocardiography
- V/Q Scan
- CT Pulmonary Angiography (+/-)
- Right Heart Catheterization
- Digital Subtraction Angiography

Serial BPA Sessions

Repeat Functional Class Assessment, NT-proBNP, 6MWT, and TTE every 3 months while BPA sessions ongoing

After either mPAP<30mmHg of all approachable lesions treated:

- Repeat WHO/NYHA Functional Class Assessment at each follow up visit
- Repeat 6MWT every 3-6 months
- Repeat TTE every 6-12 months
- Repeat Right Heart Catheterization as needed with change in functional status or symptoms

lished. Given the low cost and ease with which both evaluations can be done and their general prognostic utility, we suggest repeating the 6MWT and functional class assessment between each BPA session and at regular intervals (6–12 months) following completion of BPA treatment.

We additionally suggest that TTE be performed in follow-up after completion of BPA. As right-heart failure remains the number one cause of death in patients with CTEPH, it is important to characterize the extent of RV remodeling following treatment with BPA. TTE data is the most inconsistently reported data in the BPA literature to date for unclear reasons. In those few papers reporting RV parameters on TTE, the results have been encouraging. Several groups have reported significant improvements in various RV parame-

ters on TTE including RV mid diameter, tricuspid annular plane systolic excursion (TAPSE), RV diastolic area, and RV fractional area change (FAC) [7–9]. Interestingly in Yamagata et al.'s report on BPA in the elderly, although the classic improvements in pulmonary hemodynamics and functional capacity were observed, no significant improvements were noted in any of the RV parameters reported (RV diameter, RV FAC, and TAPSE) [34]. This discrepancy in TTE outcomes raises the question as to whether elderly patients with CTEPH are less able to achieve the RV remodeling observed in younger cohorts and warrants further investigation. Whether routine invasive assessment of hemodynamics with RHC after completion of BPA is necessary is still an area of active discussion. Most centers have opted to only repeat RHC in patients who develop worsening functional capacity or signs of worsening right-heart failure.

Nearly all BPA studies to date have utilized a similar battery of tests pre-, during, and post-BPA to characterize and report the hemodynamic and functional capacity changes associated with BPA. A small subgroup of authors, in particular those reporting novel or adjunctive modalities to improve BPA, have not reported these parameters, making the interpretation and reproducibility of their results difficult and highlighting the need for a standardized practice in workup and reporting of data within the field.

Standardization in reporting of outcomes and adverse events: As detailed above, the lack of standardization in reporting of outcomes leads to a heterogeneous field of data with differences in the magnitude of effect of BPA, difficulty with generalizability of results, and lack of clarity in actual efficacy of adjunctive modalities in treatment with BPA. Unfortunately, given the lack of prospective, randomized data in this field, it is not yet clear which endpoints are truly clinically relevant and speak to the need for dedicated studies to answer some of these questions and allow for standardization in reporting. While clinically relevant outcomes measuring the efficacy of BPA are yet to be fully defined, adverse events and procedure-related complications assessing the safety of BPA likewise need standardization in reporting.

Complications, predominantly lung injury, have been noted in a large proportion of BPA procedures since the advent of the field, occurring in as many as 61% of patients in Feinstein's initial description in 2001 [1]. Through time and refinement of the technique, complications have decreased. Two recent meta-analyses examining efficacy and safety outcomes of BPA found that the cumulative incidence of RPE was between 12.9% and 28.6% with wire injuries occurring between 5.3% and 5.6% of the time [35, 36]. Cumulative mortality was 1.9% in the short term (<30 days) and 5.7% in the long term (>30 days). As we have discussed previously in this chapter, the prevailing theory on the etiology of lung injury in BPA has shifted in recent years towards iatrogenic injury from either wire

injury, balloon over-dilation, or high-pressure contrast injection, rather than the reperfusion physiology observed in patients post-PEA. This theory is supported by the report from Ikeda et al. in 2019 which demonstrated through the use of routine CT scan immediately post-procedure in all patients undergoing BPA that lung injury was exclusively localized to the area of intervention and encompassed small areas of parenchymal opacification, as opposed to opacification of the entire area of lung perfused by a given vessel as would be expected in reperfusion injury physiology [20]. Given this shift in the understanding of BPA complications, there has been a need for an established, consensus-derived classification of complications in BPA. Inami et al. published a 5-grade classification of RPE in their seminal paper on the PEPSI-PWG method to avoid RPE [4]. Several authors through the years have utilized this scale to report their BPA-related complications. Outside of this group, there was no previously proposed standardized classification of BPA-related complications until the report by Kim et al. in 2019 [19]. This classification (Fig. 12.4) adopts the modern thought regarding the etiology of lung injury in BPA and classifies complications according to whether they occur during or after the procedure.

Centers of Excellence in CTEPH and BPA: As the field of BPA continues to grow, with the heterogeneity of reported outcomes, it is important now more than ever that we establish and recognize centers of excellence in CTEPH to ensure that patients diagnosed with CTEPH receive the best chance at a durable long-term treatment for their disease. As is noted in the diagnostic algorithm above, any patient who is suspected of having CTEPH and is found to have mismatched perfusion defects on V/Q scan should be referred to an expert CTEPH center. An expert CTEPH center previously included PEA surgeons with extensive experience, CTEPH-trained cardiothoracic radiologists, pulmonologists, and cardiologists with expertise in CTEPH. However, now with the growing presence and availability of BPA as a therapeutic option for patients with CTEPH, interventional cardiologists or radiologists with exten-

During the procedure
  Vascular injury# with/without haemoptysis
    Wire perforation
    Balloon overdilation
    High-pressure contrast injection
  Vascular dissection
  Allergic reaction to contrast
  Adverse reaction to conscious sedation/local anaesthesia
After the procedure
  Lung injury (radiographic opacity with/without haemoptysis, with/without hypoxaemia)
  Renal dysfunction
  Access site problems

#: signs of vascular injury: extravasation of contrast, hypoxaemia, cough, tachycardia, increased pulmonary arterial pressure; :causes of lung injury: vascular injury much greater than reperfusion lung injury.

Fig. 12.4 Proposed classification of BPA-related complications, as described by Kim et al. in the 2019 sixth World Symposium on Pulmonary Hypertension section on chronic thromboembolic pulmonary hypertension. Kim NH, Delcroix M, et al. Chronic Thromboembolic Pulmonary Hypertension. Eur Resp J. 2019; 53 (1):1801915

sive experience with BPA should be added to the definition of an expert CTEPH center, as this designation should include all possible therapeutic options for patients with CTEPH.

The need for high volume of PEA cases at a given center, optimally with PEA surgeons performing 50 or greater PEA surgeries per year, has been previously established [37, 38]. The advent and recognition of BPA as an alternative therapy for inoperable CTEPH patients and the wealth of data now available to us regarding the efficacy and safety profile of this therapy demand a similar expectation of the expertise of the operators performing this intervention. We have seen in the literature that those centers with the highest volume of cases have reported the lowest rates of procedure-related complications and mortality as the field has progressed. We currently lack the registry-level data utilized in PEA cohorts to determine the minimum annual case load to be considered an expert center in BPA, but this represents an opportunity for the field to grow as it defines its place in the treatment algorithm of patients with CTEPH. Further, insistence upon BPA management at CTEPH centers would ensure that patients with CTEPH are exposed to the full range of comprehensive care options including medical therapy and PEA, rather than just being treated with a potentially suboptimal BPA procedure.

12.4   Section 3: Need for Randomized Controlled Trials of BPA

To date, the vast majority of data regarding its outcomes and complications has been gleaned from either retrospective data or prospective non-comparative data, both of which have their limitations. The role BPA will ultimately play in the management of patients with inoperable CTEPH or patients with recurrent or residual PH after PEA is still evolving, particularly in relation to medical therapy. In a 2019 meta-analysis comparing riociguat with BPA by Wang et al., BPA was associated with significant improvement in mPAP, PVR, 6MWD, and functional class compared with riociguat [36]. This question of the efficacy of riociguat compared with BPA is the subject of two RCTs, the RACE study which was conducted in France and the MR BPA study being performed by investigators in Japan.

The Riociguat Versus Balloon Pulmonary Angioplasty in Non-operable Chronic ThromboEmbolic Pulmonary Hypertension (RACE) study was conducted between January 2016 and January 2019 in 14 centers in France within the French Pulmonary Hypertension Network. The study enrolled 105 patients with new diagnosis of CTEPH who were treatment-naïve and deemed to be inoperable by experienced PEA surgeons. The primary endpoint in this study was change in PVR from baseline at 26 weeks follow-up with key secondary endpoints of change in 6MWD, WHO FC, NT-pro-BNP, and time to clinical worsening. The study was completed in 2019, and preliminary results presented at the 2019 ERS International Congress indicated that BPA was superior to riociguat with respect to the primary endpoint, with a 60% reduction in the BPA group compared with 32% reduction in the riociguat arm. There was no significant difference in 6MWD between the groups, albeit with a trend towards superiority for BPA. Significantly more patients saw improvement in their WHO FC in the BPA arm compared with the riociguat arm (88% vs. 49%, p < 0.001). The full results of this trial have yet to be published.

The second ongoing RCT, the MR BPA study (UMIN000019549), is a multicenter prospective randomized controlled trial being conducted across expert BPA centers in Japan comparing BPA with riociguat, as in the RACE study. Planned enrollment is of 60 patients (30 in each arm) with diagnosis of CTEPH who are deemed non-operable for PEA. Notable exclusion criteria include prior BPA, PEA within 6 months of BPA, and pulmonary vasodilator use within 4 weeks of initial RHC. The primary endpoint in this study is change in mPAP. Secondary endpoints include change in 6MWD, WHO FC, BNP levels, TTE parameters, and importantly difference in health insurance resource cost. The length of follow-up in this study (12 months from treatment completion) is longer than that of the RACE study and may offer more nuanced information regarding hemodynamic and functional changes during the follow-up period. We eagerly await the results of the MR BPA study and the final results of the RACE study to better understand the clinical efficacy of BPA compared with riociguat.

A further lingering question has been what benefit continued therapy with pulmonary vasodilators, specifically riociguat, confers, and whether patients need to continue riociguat therapy after having completed BPA, particularly in those with normalization of their hemodynamics

post-BPA. A recent randomized open-label trial published by Aoki et al. in 2020 aimed to answer this question, at least in part [39]. Patients were randomized to either riociguat [11] or control [10] (usual medical therapy without vasodilators) after achieving hemodynamic improvement with BPA (mean mPAP = 25 mmHg in both groups). After six months of therapy, the patients underwent repeat RHC and cardiopulmonary exercise testing to assess pulmonary hemodynamics and exercise capacity. Although there was no significant difference in baseline hemodynamics between the groups, riociguat therapy resulted in significant increase in CO and decrease in PVR during exercise compared with control. This data is an excellent first step in determining the appropriate combination of BPA and pulmonary vasodilators in inoperable CTEPH patients. It is particularly helpful in that on average, the patients included had achieved normalization of their mPAP, even if not their PVR. Exercise intolerance remains the hallmark feature of patients with PH, and therefore data showing improvements in exercise tolerance and pulmonary hemodynamics with riociguat post-BPA enforce the idea that these medications may be a necessary long-term component of CTEPH care. This question bears further investigation in a larger, multicenter, multinational, placebo-controlled trial to better understand the role of riociguat post-BPA.

While these studies are a necessary and important step forward in addressing many of the unanswered questions regarding BPA, there is still much work to be done to fully understand the place of BPA within the hierarchy of medical, surgical, and interventional treatment of CTEPH. As the guidelines currently stand, riociguat is recommended first-line in all non-operable CTEPH patients. Therefore, in the modern era, most patients undergoing BPA have been on riociguat leading up to their BPA. We do not know the actual clinical benefit to this "lead-in" period with riociguat. Some have hypothesized that pretreatment with a period of riociguat prior to BPA may allow for optimization of hemodynamics prior to BPA, and, if not improve outcomes, may potentially reduce the rate of procedure-related complications. This, however, remains unproven. The notion of optimizing pulmonary hemodynamics prior to intervention in CTEPH patients with prohibitively high PVR is the subject of the ongoing PEA Bridging study (ClinicalTrials.gov Identifier: NCT03273257) comparing a 3-month pretreatment period with riociguat prior to PEA with placebo prior to PEA, and may shed light on the utility of a similar study within BPA.

As BPA technique continues to improve and expert operators are able to drive their complication and mortality rates ever lower, the question of utilizing BPA in technically operable patients is raised. In general, proximal disease involving the main, lobar, and sometimes segmental arteries has classically been felt to be surgically accessible, particularly in expert PEA centers. BPA has classically been used to address lesions in the segmental and subsegmental arteries of the pulmonary vasculature, especially for patients who are deemed non-operable strictly due to anatomic constraints (i.e., peripherally distributed CTEPH lesions). As technique and experience with PEA have advanced, expert PEA surgeons have been able to expand their field of endarterectomy out into the segmental branches of the pulmonary arteries. In this area of crossover, namely the segmental level of the pulmonary arteries, where either BPA or PEA may be a viable therapy for CTEPH, there has been no direct comparison of the two therapies. In patients who are clear surgical candidates without significant comorbidity, there is at present no question that these patients should undergo PEA as it is the only known curative intervention for CTEPH. However, in those patients with predominantly segmental disease in whom the preoperative risk profile is higher than average or with significant comorbidity that would place the patient at increased risk or peri- and postoperative complications, these patients might be better served by BPA. Several groups, predominantly in Japan, have been able to consistently achieve resolution of PH (mPAP <25 mmHg) [3, 23, 40–42]. In a recent systematic review and meta-analysis comparing the safety and efficacy of BPA, PEA, and medical therapy, there was no difference in 2-year mortality between PEA and BPA, while BPA outperformed medical therapy in 6MWD, improvements in pulmonary hemodynamics, and WHO FC [43]. If the field of BPA is able to consistently obtain the level of hemodynamic improvement and normalization achieved in PEA, a randomized controlled trial comparing BPA to PEA in patients with segmental predominant disease would be reasonable and useful to better define the role of BPA in this population.

12.5 Section 4: Long-Term Follow-up Data

The young age of the field of BPA, having only been rejuvenated in the last decade, makes long-term outcome data scarce in the BPA literature. There have been no reports of longer term outcomes to allow for more direct comparison of the durability of hemodynamic effects, safety, and functional capacity with PEA. Existent data for short- and midterm mortality are promising, including reports from Japan with 98.5–100% 2-year survival, 94.5% 2-year survival in a Polish cohort, and 95.1% 3-year survival in the French cohort which are all comparable with PEA [3, 5, 6, 12]. The longest term outcome data we have to date is from Aoki et al. with a 98.4% survival rate at 5 years in 77 patients who underwent BPA [40]. Survival data is important but functional outcomes must also be considered. In addition, it would be useful to know if the hemodynamic effects of BPA have comparable durability to those of PEA. Further, functional outcome data will allow clinicians to manage patient expectations appropriately and more adequately prognosticate their clinical course. One of the methods to generate this data would be the formation of a multinational consortium to share and pool data akin to those that exist in the field of PEA. A central repository of BPA data would allow for more robust analyses that can be generalized to a larger proportion of the field.

12.6 Conclusion

Over the last decade BPA has emerged as a potential therapy option for a select group of CTEPH patients. Continued refinement in patient selection, anatomic consideration, operator technique, and long-term follow-up has the potential to improve the safety and efficacy of BPA, ensuring that it is used appropriately, with the goal of achieving improved outcomes for patients with CTEPH.

References

 1. Feinstein JA, Goldhaber SZ, et al. Balloon pulmonary angioplasty for treatment of chronic thromboembolic pulmonary hypertension. Circulation. 2001;103(1):10–3.
 2. Kataoka M, Inami T, et al. Percutaneous transluminal pulmonary angioplasty for the treatment of chronic thromboembolic pulmonary hypertension. Circ Cardiovasc Interv. 2012;5(6):756–62.
 3. Mizoguchi H, Ogawa A, Munemasa M, Mikouchi H, Matsubara H. Refined balloon pulmonary angioplasty for inoperable patients with chronic thromboembolic pulmonary hypertension. Circ Cardiovasc Interv. 2012;5(6):748–55.
 4. Inami T, Kataoka M, et al. Pulmonary edema predictive scoring index (PEPSI), a new index to predict risk of reperfusion pulmonary edema and improvement of hemodynamics in percutaneous transluminal pulmonary angioplasty. JACC Cardiovasc Interv. 2013;6(7):725–36.
 5. Szymon D, Kurzyna M, Pietura R, Torbicki A. Balloon pulmonary angioplasty for inoperable chronic thromboembolic pulmonary hypertension. Kardiol Pol. 2013;71(12):1331.
 6. Brenot P, Jaïs X, et al. French experience of balloon pulmonary angioplasty for chronic thromboembolic pulmonary hypertension. Eur Respir J. 2019;53(5):1802095.
 7. Olsson KM, Wiedenroth CB, el. Balloon pulmonary angioplasty for inoperable chronic thromboembolic pulmonary hypertension: the initial German experience. Eur Respir J. 2017;49(6):1602409.
 8. Anand V, Frantz RP, et al. Balloon pulmonary angioplasty for chronic thromboembolic pulmonary hypertension: initial single-center experience. Mayo Clin Proc Innov Qual Outcomes. 2019;3(3):311–8.
 9. Hoole SP, Coghlan JG, et al. Balloon pulmonary angioplasty for inoperable chronic thromboembolic pulmonary hypertension: the UK experience. Open Heart. 2020;7(1):e001144.
10. Andreassen AK, Ragnarsson A, Gude E, Geiran O, Andersen R. Balloon pulmonary angioplasty in patients with inoperable chronic thromboembolic pulmonary hypertension. Heart. 2013;99(19):1415–20.
11. Godinas L, Bonne L, et al. Balloon pulmonary angioplasty for the treatment of nonoperable chronic thromboembolic pulmonary hypertension: single-center experience with low initial complication rate. J Vasc Interv Radiol. 2019;30(8):1265–72.
12. Hinrichs JB, Marquardt S, et al. Comparison of C-arm computed tomography and digital subtraction angiography in patients with chronic thromboembolic pulmonary hypertension. Cardiovasc Intervent Radiol. 2016;39(1):53–63.
13. Maschke SK, Hinrichs JB, et al. C-arm computed tomography (CACT)-guided balloon pulmonary angioplasty (BPA): evaluation of patient safety and peri- and post-procedural complications. Eur Radiol. 2019;29(3):1276–84.
14. Nagayoshi S, Fujii S, Nakajima T, Muto M. Intravenous ultrasound-guided balloon pulmonary angioplasty in the treatment of totally occluded chronic thromboembolic pulmonary hypertension. EuroIntervention. 2018;14(2):234–5.
15. Lin JL, Chen HM, et al. Application of DynaCT angiographic reconstruction in balloon pulmonary angioplasty. Eur Radiol. 2020;30(12):6950–7.
16. Roik M, Wretowski D, et al. Refined balloon pulmonary angioplasty driven by combined assessment of intra-arterial anatomy and physiology—multimodal approach to treated lesions in patients with non-operable distal chronic thromboembolic pulmonary hypertension—technique, safety, and efficacy of 50 consecutive angioplasties. Int J Cardiol. 2016;203:228–35.
17. Hinrichs JB, Renne J, et al. Balloon pulmonary angioplasty: applicability of C-arm CT for procedure guidance. Eur Radiol. 2016;26(11):4064–71.
18. Maschke SK, Winther HMB, et al. Evaluation of a newly developed 2D parametric parenchymal blood flow technique with an automated vessel suppression algorithm in patients with chronic thromboembolic pulmonary hypertension undergoing balloon pulmonary angioplasty. Clin Radiol. 2019;74(6):437–44.
19. Kim NH, Delcroix M, et al. Chronic thromboembolic pulmonary hypertension. Eur Respir J. 2019;53(1):1801915.
20. Ikeda N, Kubota S, et al. The predictors of complications in balloon pulmonary angioplasty for chronic thromboembolic pulmonary hypertension. Catheter Cardiovasc Interv. 2019;93(6):e349–56.
21. Kawakami T, Ogawa A, et al. Novel angiographic classification of each vascular lesion in chronic thromboembolic pulmonary hypertension based on selective angiogram and results of balloon pulmonary angioplasty. Circ Cardiovasc Interv. 2016;9(10):e003318.
22. Kurzyna M, Darocha S, et al. Changing the strategy of balloon pulmonary angioplasty resulted in a reduced complication rate in patients with chronic thromboembolic pulmonary hypertension. A single center European experience. Kardiol Pol. 2017;75(7):645–54.

23. Ogawa A, Satoh T, et al. Balloon pulmonary angioplasty for chronic thromboembolic pulmonary hypertension: results of a multicenter registry. Circ Cardiovasc Qual Outcomes. 2017;10(11):e004029.

24. Kawakami T, Kataoka M, et al. Retrograde approach in balloon pulmonary angioplasty: useful novel strategy for chronic Total occlusion lesions in pulmonary arteries. JACC Cardiovasc Interv. 2016;9(2):e19–20.

25. Kawashima T, Yoshitake A, Kawakami T, Shimizu H. Two-stage treatment using balloon pulmonary angioplasty and pulmonary endarterectomy in a patient with chronic thromboembolic pulmonary hypertension. Ann Vasc Surg. 2018;49:315.e5–7.

26. Wiedenroth CB, Liebetrau C, et al. Combined pulmonary endarterectomy and balloon pulmonary angioplasty in patients with chronic thromboembolic pulmonary hypertension. J Heart Lung Transplatn. 2016;35(5):591–6.

27. Araszkiewicz A, Darocha S, et al. Balloon pulmonary angioplasty for the treatment of residual or recurrent pulmonary hypertension after pulmonary endarterectomy. Int J Cardiol. 2019;278:232–7.

28. Shimura N, Kataoka M, et al. Additional percutaneous transluminal pulmonary angioplasty for residual of recurrent pulmonary hypertension after pulmonary endarterectomy. Int J Cardiol. 2015;183:138–42.

29. Yanaka K, Nakayama K, et al. Sequential hybrid therapy with pulmonary endarterectomy and balloon pulmonary angioplasty for chronic thromboembolic pulmonary hypertension. J Am Heart Assoc. 2018;7(13):e008838.

30. Galiè N, Humbert M, et al. 2015 ESC/ERS guidelines for the diagnosis and treatment of pulmonary hypertension: the joint taskforce for the diagnosis and treatment of pulmonary hypertension of the European Society of Cardiology (ESC) and the European Respiratory Society (ERS): endorsed by: Association for European Paediatric and Congenital Cardiology (AEPC), International Society for Heart and Lung Transplantation (ISHLT). Eur Respir J. 2015;46(4):903–75.

31. Ghofrani HA, D'Armini AM, et al. Riociguat for the treatment of chronic thromboembolic pulmonary hypertension. N Engl J Med. 2013;369(4):319–29.

32. Simonneau G, D'Armini AM, et al. Riociguat for the treatment of chronic thromboembolic pulmonary hypertension: a long-term extension study (CHEST-2). Eur Respir J. 2015;45(5):1293–302.

33. Souza R, Channick RN, et al. Association between six-minute walk distance and long-term outcomes in patients and pulmonary arterial hypertension: data from the randomized SERAPHIN trial. PLoS One. 2018;13(3):e0193226.

34. Yamagata Y, Ikeda S, et al. Balloon pulmonary angioplasty is effective for treating peripheral-type chronic thromboembolic pulmonary hypertension in elderly patients. Geriatr Gerontol Int. 2018;18(5):678–84.

35. Kalra R, Duval S, et al. Comparison of balloon pulmonary angioplasty and pulmonary vasodilators for inoperable chronic thromboembolic pulmonary hypertension: a systematic review and meta-analysis. Sci Rep. 2020;10(1):8870.

36. Wang W, Wen L, Song Z, Shi W, Wang K, Huang W. Balloon pulmonary angioplasty vs. Riociguat in patients with inoperable chronic thromboembolic pulmonary hypertension: a systematic review and meta-analysis. Clin Cardiol. 2019;42(8):741–52.

37. Cannon JE, Su L, et al. Dynamic risk stratification of patient long-term outcome after pulmonary endarterectomy: results from the United Kingdom National Cohort. Circulation. 2016;133(18):1761–71.

38. Jenkins D, Madani M, Fadel E, D'Armini AM, Mayer E. Pulmonary endarterectomy for the treatment of chronic thromboembolic pulmonary hypertension. Eur Respir Rev. 2017;26(143):160111.

39. Aoki T, Sugimura K, et al. Beneficial effects of Riociguat on hemodynamic responses to exercise in CTEPH patients after balloon pulmonary angioplasty—a randomized controlled study. Int J Cardiol Heart Vasc. 2020;29:100579.

40. Aoki T, Sugimura K, et al. Comprehensive evaluation of the effectiveness and safety of balloon pulmonary angioplasty for inoperable chronic thrombo-embolic pulmonary hypertension: long-term effects and procedure-related complications. Eur Heart J. 2017;38(42):3152–9.

41. Kimura M, Kohno T, et al. Midterm effect of balloon pulmonary angioplasty on hemodynamics and subclinical myocardial damage in chronic thromboembolic pulmonary hypertension. Can J Cardiol. 2017;33(4):463–70.

42. Taniguchi Y, Miyagawa K, et al. Balloon pulmonary angioplasty: an additional treatment option to improve the prognosis of patients with chronic thromboembolic pulmonary hypertension. EuroIntervention. 2014;10(4):518–25.

43. Tanabe N, Kawakami T, et al. Balloon pulmonary angioplasty for chronic thromboembolic pulmonary hypertension: a systematic review. Respir Investig. 2018;56(4):332–41.

Chronic Thromboembolic Pulmonary Hypertension and Chronic Thromboembolic Pulmonary Disease (CTEPD): Clinical and Interventional Perspective

13

Fabio Dardi, Massimiliano Palazzini, Daniele Guarino, Nevio Taglieri, Alessandra Manes, Nazzareno Galiè, and Francesco Saia

Abbreviations

6MWD	6-min walk distance
BMI	Body mass index
BPA	Balloon pulmonary angioplasty
CPET	Cardiopulmonary exercise testing
CT	Computed tomography
CTEPD	Chronic thromboembolic pulmonary disease
CTEPH	Chronic thromboembolic pulmonary hypertension
DECT	Dual-energy computed tomography angiography
DOAC	Direct oral anticoagulant
mPAP	Mean pulmonary artery pressure
NT-proBNP	N-terminal pro-brain natriuretic peptide
P/Q	Pressure/flow (mPAP/cardiac output)
PE	Pulmonary embolism
PEA	Pulmonary endarterectomy
PH	Pulmonary hypertension
PVR	Pulmonary vascular resistance
RHC	Right-heart catheterization
RV	Right ventricle
sPAP	Systolic pulmonary arterial pressure
V/Q	Ventilation/perfusion
VE/VCO$_2$	Minute ventilation/carbon dioxide production
VO$_2$	Oxygen uptake
VTE	Venous thromboembolism

F. Dardi (✉) · M. Palazzini · D. Guarino · N. Taglieri · A. Manes · N. Galiè · F. Saia
Cardiology Unit, Cardio-Thoracic-Vascular Department, IRCCS University Hospital of Bologna, Policlinico S. Orsola, Bologna, Italy
e-mail: fabio.dardi@aosp.bo.it;
massimiliano.palazzini@unibo.it;
daniele.guarino3@unibo.it; nevio.taglieri@aosp.bo.it;
alessandra.manes@unibo.it; nazzareno.galie@unibo.it;
francesco.saia@unibo.it

© Springer Nature Switzerland AG 2022
F. Saia et al. (eds.), *Balloon pulmonary angioplasty in patients with CTEPH*,
https://doi.org/10.1007/978-3-030-95997-5_13

13.1 Definition of Chronic Thromboembolic Pulmonary Disease (CTEPD)

Chronic thromboembolic pulmonary disease (CTEPD) is characterized by symptoms and perfusion defects similar to chronic thromboembolic pulmonary hypertension (CTEPH), after at least 3 months of adequate anticoagulation treatment, but without pulmonary hypertension (PH) at rest [1, 2]. Current European Society of Cardiology (ESC)/European Respiratory Society (ERS) guidelines define CTEPH as the presence of precapillary PH [mean pulmonary artery pressure (mPAP) $\geq$25 mmHg and pulmonary artery wedge pressure (PAWP) $\leq$15 mmHg], together with mismatched perfusion defects on lung scan and specific diagnostic signs seen by multidetector CT angiography, MR imaging, or conventional pulmonary angiography, such as ringlike stenosis, webs/slits, wall irregularities, and chronic total occlusions [3]. Recently, a new threshold for PH [mPAP >20 mmHg] and precapillary PH [combination of mPAP >20 mmHg, PAWP $\leq$15 mmHg, and pulmonary vascular resistance (PVR) $\geq$3 Wood units (WU)] has been proposed by the sixth World Symposium on PH [4]. The consequences of this new definition for CTEPH and CTEPD are not yet established. It is worthwhile to underline that in patients with perfusion defects and mild elevation of mPAP (20–24 mmHg), PVR is generally >3 WU so a mPAP of 20 mmHg seems indicative of a significant pulmonary vascular disease in patients with

group 4 PH [5]. A tentative, comprehensive definition of CTEPD has been recently proposed by the Task Force on CTEPH during the sixth World Symposium on PH (Table 13.1).

13.2 Epidemiology of CTEPD

CTEPD is increasingly encountered in pulmonary vascular disease clinics following acute pulmonary embolism (PE) and its incidence is going to increase also thanks to the clinical awareness aroused by the latest ESC/ERS PE guidelines. As a matter of fact, according to these guidelines, all acute PE survivors should undergo a systematic follow-up evaluation at 3–6 months to detect the presence of dyspnea or functional limitation. This means that a significant number of patients should seek medical attention as self-reported dyspnea and measured poor physical performance are present in more than 50% of the patients 6 months to 3 years after adequately treated acute PE in most case series [6]. Dyspnea and reduced effort tolerance anyway are not the only symptoms reported: in the study of Dzikowska-Diduch et al. 65% of 845 acute PE survivors reported significant functional limitation, in particular 33% had exertional dyspnea, 12% had effort angina, 6% had palpitations, and 49% complained about reduced exercise tolerance. Predictors of exertional dyspnea at long-term follow-up after acute PE are advanced age, cardiac or pulmonary comorbidities, high body mass index (BMI), history of smoking, high pul-

Table 13.1 CTEPD compared with CTEPH (adapted from Kim et al [1])

Diagnostic criteria	CTEPH	CTEPD
Symptoms	Exercise dyspnea	Exercise dyspnea
PH	Present at rest	Absent at rest
RHC at exercise		P/Q slope > 3 mmHg·l^{-1}·min^{-1}
V/Q scan	Any mismatched perfusion defect	Any mismatched perfusion defect
Angio-CT scan	Typical findings of CTEPH	Typical findings of CTEPH
CPET		Excluding ventilatory limitation, deconditioning
Transthoracic echocardiogram		Excluding left-heart disease
Anticoagulation	At least 3 months	At least 3 months

CPET cardiopulmonary exercise test, *CT* computed tomography, *CTEPH* chronic thromboembolic pulmonary hypertension, *PH* pulmonary hypertension, *P/Q* pressure/flow, *RHC* right-heart catheterization, *V/Q* ventilation/perfusion.

monary artery systolic pressure (sPAP) and right ventricular (RV) dysfunction at diagnosis, and residual pulmonary vascular obstruction at discharge [7]. Predictors of reduced peak oxygen uptake (VO$_2$) at cardiopulmonary exercise testing (CPET) at 1-year follow-up are male sex, advanced age, high BMI, current or previous smoking status, percent predicted peak VO$_2$ < 80% at 1 month, and reduced 6-minute walk distance (6MWD) at 1 month [8]. Eventually, predictors of reduced exercise capacity and quality of life over time included female sex, high BMI, history of lung disease, high sPAP, and high main pulmonary artery diameter at CT scan [9].

It is important to underline that the complete resolution of thrombi may be achieved in 70–85% of patients 6–12 months after an acute PE diagnosis with partial resolution in the vast majority of the remaining patients. Larger and more centrally located blood clots, older age, longer duration of symptoms before PE diagnosis, and history of venous thromboembolism (VTE) are associated with a lower degree of thrombus resolution [10].

Taken together, these data suggest that muscle deconditioning, particularly in the presence of excess body weight and cardiopulmonary comorbidities, is largely responsible for the frequently reported dyspnea and exercise limitation after acute PE rather than the mere presence of residual thrombi or persisting/progressive PH and RV dysfunction. As a matter of fact according to Dzikowska-Diduch et al. the causes of the persistence of symptoms after an acute PE were left ventricular diastolic dysfunction (34.2%), chronic obstructive pulmonary disease (9.3%), coronary artery disease (6.9%), reduced left ventricular ejection fraction (6.9%), atrial fibrillation (6.9%), and left ventricular valvular disease (6.2%), and only 8.4% (4.5% of all survivors) of patients were finally diagnosed as CTEPH and 3.3% with CTEPD [7].

Also in light of these data, transthoracic echocardiogram must be considered the first-line evaluation in PE patients' follow-up (as it is able to highlight the actual impairment of RV function and to detect signs of left heart disease) and it should be performed, assessing also

the probability of PH (thus possible CTEPH), in patients complaining dyspnea and/or poor physical performance but may be considered also in patients with risk factors for CTEPH. Patients with a high echocardiographic probability of PH, or those with intermediate probability combined with elevated N-terminal pro-brain natriuretic peptide (NT-proBNP) levels, risk factors for CTEPH, or abnormal results at CPET, should undergo ventilation/perfusion (V/Q) lung scintigraphy to detect mismatched perfusion defects in order to evaluate the referral of the patient to a PH expert center for further diagnostic workup [6].

13.3 CTEPD Pathophysiology: Exercise Cardiopulmonary and Hemodynamic Characteristics

The pathophysiologic processes involved in the development of CTEPD after acute PE are incompletely understood. For sure, after an acute PE one or more pulmonary emboli fail to resolve through fibrinolysis leading to chronic obstruction of the pulmonary vascular bed but the process may not be so simple. The reasons why some patients develop PH and some may not can be that in the latter the number of occluded segments is insufficient to affect resistance at rest but also that no secondary vasculopathy has developed. The role of secondary vasculopathy can be inferred by the fact that, if simple obstruction is the only issue, pulmonary endarterectomy (PEA) should lead to complete resolution of PH in all cases of CTEPH but this does not occur. Anyway, whether the trigger for a vasculopathy development (intimal and medial hypertrophy in unaffected sub-500 μm vessels) is primarily related to the degree of vascular obstruction or to individual patient factors predisposing them to PH is unresolved. Thus, understanding the pathophysiology remains of pivotal importance to early detect CTEPD and its possible progression to CTEPH.

By definition in CTEPD hemodynamics at rest is within the normal limits. The main instrumental tests that allow to analyze the pathophysiology of the pulmonary circulation during physical exercise are the CPET and the exercise right-heart catheterization. Technical and procedural aspects of these two techniques have been recently reviewed in patients with PH [4, 11].

Claeys et al. evaluated 14 CTEPD patients in comparison with 13 healthy volunteers to understand the factors that limit exercise capacity in patients with persistent pulmonary artery obstructions. Compared to control subjects, patients with CTEPD had a worse performance at CPET (lower peak VO_2, peak power, peak heart rate, and peak respiratory exchange ratio) and different RV adaptation at exercise: RV end-diastolic and end-systolic volume did not decline with exercise, stroke volume and RV ejection fraction were lower and increased less through the duration of exercise, RV contractility is higher at rest but RV contractile reserve is lower and pulmonary arterial compliance is lower both at baseline and at peak exercise. Moreover, peak VO_2 seems more closely related to RV contractile reserve, cardiac output, mPAP/cardiac output (P/Q) slope, and minute ventilation/carbon dioxide production (VE/VCO_2) rather than dead space ventilation. These data suggest that patients with CTEPD have a subtle increase in pulmonary vascular load that can be compensated at rest by an increased RV contractility (to maintain ventricular-arterial coupling) but is unmasked during exercise and can be, at least in part, an explanation of CTEPD patients' symptoms [12]. This can be inferred also by the fact that occult RV dysfunction can be unmasked by ventricular-arterial coupling analysis: CTEPD patients with lower ventricular-arterial coupling have a higher VE/VCO_2 slope [13] and have a "left ventricularization" of pressure-volume loop morphology [patients with CTEPD continue to develop RV pressure during systolic ejection similarly to CTEPH patients in whom increased resistance and lower arterial compliance are exposed to the RV early after pulmonary valve opening (RV end-systolic pressure > RV pressure at the time of pulmonary valve opening) differently from healthy subjects in whom there is a rapid dissipation in pressure during systole with ejection into a more compliant pulmonary circulation (RV end-systolic pressure < RV pressure at the time of pulmonary valve opening)] [14].

Van Kan et al. confirm that patients with CTEPD have an increased VE/VCO_2 but they observed also a nonphysiological increase in dead space ventilation during exercise, especially in patients with a steep P/Q slope and lower pulmonary arterial compliance. Nine patients with a mPAP >30 mmHg at peak exercise underwent PEA after which there was an increase of peak workload and VO_2, a decrease of dead space ventilation, and normalization of VE/VCO_2 [15]. So, despite some discrepancies between the studies it can be hypothesized that chronic thrombi do affect gas exchange just as acute thrombi: the presence of vascular occlusions can limit perfusion of the alveolar units dependent on these vessels and lead to ventilation/perfusion imbalance and ventilatory inefficiency, which is more evident during exercise [10].

Dead space ventilation, anyway, is much higher in patients with CTEPH compared to CTEPD patients and has been proposed as a predictor of PH at rest in patients with pulmonary thromboembolic obstructions independently from the degree of proximal thrombotic burden [16].

Regarding hemodynamic characteristics, Guth et al. evaluated 12 CTEPD patients with exercise hemodynamic before and 1 year after PEA. Nine patients have a P/Q slope > 3 WU and, among them, all but one (who had an increase of pulmonary arterial wedge pressure) have a decrease of P/Q slope below 3 WU after PEA. After PEA there was also a significant improvement of peak workload and VO_2, VE/VCO_2, O_2 pulse, and symptoms [17]. From a pathophysiological point of view a steep P/Q slope is due to a lower capacity for recruitment and distension of the pulmonary vascular bed as an adaptation mechanism to the increase in stroke volume that occurs during exercise. This reduced pulmonary arterial compliance (defined as stroke volume/pulse pressure) determines an increase in the afterload of the right ventricle that leads to a decreased stroke volume (and an increase in the compensatory chronotropic response), an increased pulse pressure and, thus, an increased mPAP (defined as diastolic pulmonary arterial pressure + 1/3 of pulse pressure).

Another aspect to be considered is the localization of pulmonary artery thrombi: impedance to pulmonary forward flow may be markedly different between patients with proximal versus distal lesions, with a greater effect on RV afterload arising from proximal pulmonary vascular obstructions. Discrimination between proximal thrombus on angio-computed tomography (CT) scan and more distal obstruction on scintigraphy may, therefore, be important in defining the hemodynamic effect of CTEPD, and its impact on RV function and symptoms [18].

13.4   CTEPD Imaging

Incomplete resolution and recanalization of acute emboli result in laminated thrombi, single bands parallel to the vessel (shelves) or multiple bands in a complex weblike network, as well as complete vascular occlusions. While pulmonary angio-CT scan has almost replaced V/Q scan for the diagnosis of acute PE, V/Q scan remains the reference imaging in the workup for CTEPD as showed for CTEPH in Chap. 2. As a matter of fact a normal V/Q scan definitively excludes CTEPD with a sensitivity of 90–100% and specificity of 94–100% [3] even if its accuracy is limited in the setting of chronic lung disease or other comorbidities that affect baseline ventilation and/or perfusion or of nonocclusive thrombi with underestimation of disease extent. The main issue of angio-CT in CTEPD setting is that it must be read by an experienced cardiothoracic radiologist because it has a lower diagnostic accuracy in many lower volume settings with a sensitivity and a specificity of 76% and 96%, respectively [19]. More precisely, a recent study showed that sensitivity, specificity, and accuracy were above 90% for both V/Q scan and angio-CT but at segmental level V/Q scan is more sensitive than angio-CT (85% vs. 67%) but less specific (42% vs. 60%) [20]. Anyway, angio-CT is fundamental for delineation of the

extent of thrombus burden and to guide therapeutic decision-making. Ideally, the optimal technique would allow for an assessment of the pulmonary arterial tree and provide a reliable evaluation of lung perfusion in one sitting and dual-energy computed tomography angiography (DECT) and iodine subtraction mapping can be potential solutions with promising results. Recently, DECT small- and moderate-sized studies have shown a diagnostic accuracy similar to that of V/Q scintigraphy [21] and there is an ongoing study evaluating the diagnostic performance of computed tomography lung subtraction iodine mapping in comparison with V/Q scan and angio-CT [22].

13.5   Treatment

13.5.1   Anticoagulation

According to current ESC/ERS guidelines on PH, anticoagulation in CTEPH is prescribed under a class 1 recommendation. Someone extrapolated from these guidelines the recourse to extended anticoagulation also in CTEPD [3]. However, when CTEPD is diagnosed after an index acute PE associated with a major transient risk factor, uncertainties arise, the decision to extend anticoagulation may not automatically apply, and definitive anticoagulation recommendations will be lacking [18]. Regarding the choice of anticoagulation it is worthwhile to cite the study of Bunclark et al. enrolling 1000 patients following PEA: post-PEA functional and hemodynamic outcomes appear unaffected by anticoagulant choice but, differently from the studies on direct oral anticoagulants (DOACs) in acute PE, in this chronic setting bleeding events were similar and recurrent VTE rates were significantly higher in those receiving DOACs in comparison with vitamin K antagonist-treated patients [23]. So, even the choice of the best type and of the optimal dose of the anticoagulant in CTEPD patients can be problematic, especially several months after the index acute PE event as evidences are scarce.

13.5.2 Pulmonary Endarterectomy (PEA)

No controlled trials have been performed for PEA in CTEPD patients and what we know today derives only from cohort studies. In particular:

- Swietlik et al.: Among 34 patients with CTEPD 6 symptomatic patients received surgical treatment while the others were followed up for 1 year. Operated patients had hemodynamic, symptomatic, and functional improvement and none of them died; instead nonsurgically treated patients remained symptomatic but clinically and objectively stable and 2 of them died for malignancy [24].
- Van Kan et al.: 9 symptomatic CTEPD patients underwent PEA obtaining an increase of peak workload and VO_2, a decrease of dead space ventilation, and normalization of VE/VCO_2. None of them died and postoperative course was unremarkable in all [15].
- Guth et al.: 12 symptomatic CTEPD patients underwent PEA with a significant decrease of P/Q slope and improvement of peak workload, VO_2, VE/VCO_2, O_2 pulse, and symptoms. All survived the perioperative period but 3 had complications: 1 urinary tract infection, 1 atrial fibrillation, and 1 postoperative seizure and need of tracheostomy [17].
- Donahoe et al.: 14 symptomatic CTEPD patients experienced, after PEA, a significant improvement of mPAP, total pulmonary resistance, and symptoms. Perioperative mortality was 0% but there were 2 complications (pneumonia and tracheostomy). In this case series 1 patient with CTEPD treated conservatively eventually progressed to CTEPH and required lung transplantation, suggesting that this risk, albeit potentially small, can be real [25].
- Yıldızeli et al.: 23 symptomatic CTEPD patients underwent PEA with a significant improvement of mPAP, PVR, symptoms, and 6MWD. There was no in-hospital mortality, but 6 patients had complications after PEA: 2 supraventricular arrhythmias requiring cardioversion, 1 difficult weaning requiring tracheostomy, 1 cardiac tamponade, 1 reversible acute kidney injury requiring hemodialysis, and 1 transient vocal cord paralysis. Two patients died after discharge (1 for myocardial infarction and 1 for sudden death) [26].
- Taboada et al.: 42 symptomatic CTEPD patients underwent PEA with a significant improvement of mPAP, PVR, symptoms, and 6MWD. There was no in-hospital mortality, but 17 patients had major complications: 3 returned to operating theatre for cardiac tamponade, hemothorax, and supraventricular tachycardia with low cardiac output; 4 pneumothoraxes; 6 small subdural hematomas; 3 re-intubations; and 1 tracheostomy. Two patients died after discharge: 1 PE recurrence and 1 sudden death [27].

13.5.3 Balloon Pulmonary Angioplasty (BPA)

No controlled trials have been performed for BPA in CTEPD patients and what we know today derives only from cohort studies. In particular it is worthwhile to cite 2 case series:

- Wiedenroth et al.: 10 symptomatic CTEPD patients underwent BPA (the median number of sessions/patients was 4, and the median number of vessels treated/patient was 10) with a significant improvement of pulmonary arterial compliance, PVR, and symptoms. No patients died during the follow-up period and there was one wire perforation of the pulmonary vasculature with mild hemoptysis not requiring intervention [28].
- Inami et al.: 15 symptomatic CTEPD patients underwent BPA (the median number of sessions/patients was 2, and the median number of vessels treated/patient was 9) with a significant improvement of mPAP, PVR, and 6MWD. The exercise hemodynamics performed in 6 patients after BPA demonstrated a significant reduction of mPAP and PVR at peak exercise and a significant reduction in mean P/Q slope that went to values <3 WU in all patients. CPET demonstrated a significant improvement of VE/VCO_2 slope. No patients

died during the follow-up period and there were no occurrences of reperfusion pulmonary edema or pulmonary injuries across the sessions [29].

Regarding surgical and interventional treatment of CTEPD, although the case series published show an improvement of symptoms, exercise and functional capacity, and hemodynamic profile, some critical issues remain unsolved: in particular 1) the proportion of patients that remain breathless after an acute PE because of the consequences of thromboembolic disease and not because of comorbid diseases; 2) the natural history of CTEPD and how many patients will develop CTEPH or will exhibit a higher event rate during follow-up; and 3) the role of surgical/interventional treatment in altering the natural history or at least improving symptoms of CTEPD in sham-controlled studies.

In light of these considerations all interventions with both PEA and BPA should be applied only after careful balancing of benefits and risks. As a matter of fact, PEA seems to have a very low in-hospital mortality in CTEPD patients but up to 30–40% of patients may experience complications; BPA is a complex, prolonged procedure associated with significant radiation exposure and a not negligible complication rate and the reported low per-procedure complication rate in patients without PH has to be demonstrated in an adequately sized population. At present, patients with CTEPD urgently need a better understanding of their disorder in order to accordingly evaluate the best management and therapeutic algorithm; up to now, CTEPH treatment guidelines should not be applied to CTEPD [1, 30].

References

1. Kim NH, Delcroix M, Jais X, Madani MM, Matsubara H, Mayer E, Ogo T, Tapson VF, Ghofrani HA, Jenkins DP. Chronic thromboembolic pulmonary hypertension. Eur Respir J. 2019;53:1801915.
2. Delcroix M, Torbicki A, Gopalan D, Sitbon O, Klok FA, Lang I, Jenkins D, Kim NH, Humbert M, Jais X, Noordegraaf AV, Pepke-Zaba J, Brénot P, Dorfmuller P, Fadel E, Ghofrani H-A, Hoeper MM, Jansa P, Madani M, Matsubara H, Ogo T, Grünig E, D'Armini A, Galie N, Meyer B, Corkery P, Meszaros G, Mayer E, Simonneau G. ERS statement on chronic thromboembolic pulmonary hypertension. Eur Respir J. 2020;57:2002828.
3. Galiè N, Humbert M, Vachiery J-L, Gibbs S, Lang I, Torbicki A, Simonneau G, Peacock A, Vonk Noordegraaf A, Beghetti M, Ghofrani A, Gomez Sanchez MA, Hansmann G, Klepetko W, Lancellotti P, Matucci M, McDonagh T, Pierard LA, Trindade PT, Zompatori M, Hoeper M, Vachiéry J-L, Gibbs S, Lang I, Torbicki A, Simonneau G, Peacock A, Vonk-Noordegraaf A, Beghetti M, Ghofrani A, Gomez Sanchez MA, Hansmann G, Klepetko W, Lancellotti P, Matucci M, McDonagh T, Pierard LA, Trindade PT, Zompatori M, Hoeper M, Vachiery J-L, Gibbs S, Lang I, Torbicki A, Simonneau G, Peacock A, Vonk Noordegraaf A, Beghetti M, Ghofrani A, Gomez Sanchez MA, Hansmann G, Klepetko W, Lancellotti P, Matucci M, McDonagh T, Pierard LA, Trindade PT, Zompatori M, Hoeper M. 2015 ESC/ERS guidelines for the diagnosis and treatment of pulmonary hypertension. Eur Heart J. 2015;37:67–119.
4. Simonneau G, Montani D, Celermajer DS, Denton CP, Gatzoulis MA, Krowka M, Williams PG, Souza R. Haemodynamic definitions and updated clinical classification of pulmonary hypertension. Eur Respir J. 2019;53:1801913.
5. Pepke-Zaba J, Delcroix M, Lang I, Mayer E, Jansa P, Ambroz D, Treacy C, D'Armini AM, Morsolini M, Snijder R, Bresser P, Torbicki A, Kristensen B, Lewczuk J, Simkova I, Barberà JA, De Perrot M, Hoeper MM, Gaine S, Speich R, Gomez-Sanchez MA, Kovacs G, Hamid AM, Jaïs X, Simonneau G. Chronic thromboembolic pulmonary hypertension (CTEPH): results from an international prospective registry. Circulation. 2011;124:1973–81.
6. Konstantinides SV, Meyer G, Becattini C, Bueno H, Geersing G-J, Harjola V-P, Huisman MV, Humbert M, Jennings CS, Jiménez D, Kucher N, Lang IM, Lankeit M, Lorusso R, Mazzolai L, Meneveau N, Ní Áinle F, Prandoni P, Pruszczyk P, Righini M, Torbicki A, Van Belle E, Zamorano JL, ESC Scientific Document Group. 2019 ESC guidelines for the diagnosis and management of acute pulmonary embolism developed in collaboration with the European Respiratory Society (ERS). Eur Heart J. 2020;41:543–603.
7. Dzikowska-Diduch O, Kostrubiec M, Kurnicka K, Lichodziejewska B, Pacho S, Miroszewska A, Bródka K, Skowrońska M, Łabyk A, Roik M, Gołębiowski M, Pruszczyk P. The post-pulmonary syndrome - results of echocardiographic driven follow up after acute pulmonary embolism. Thromb Res. 2020;186:30–5.
8. Kahn SR, Hirsch AM, Akaberi A, Hernandez P, Anderson DR, Wells PS, Rodger MA, Solymoss S, Kovacs MJ, Rudski L, Shimony A, Dennie C, Rush C, Geerts WH, Aaron SD, Granton JT. Functional and exercise limitations after a first episode of pulmonary

embolism: results of the ELOPE prospective cohort study. Chest. 2017;151:1058–68.

9. Kahn SR, Akaberi A, Granton JT, Anderson DR, Wells PS, Rodger MA, Solymoss S, Kovacs MJ, Rudski L, Shimony A, Dennie C, Rush C, Hernandez P, Aaron SD, Hirsch AM. Quality of life, dyspnea, and functional exercise capacity following a first episode of pulmonary embolism: results of the ELOPE cohort study. Am J Med. 2017;130:990.

10. Klok FA, van der Hulle T, den Exter PL, Lankeit M, Huisman MV, Konstantinides S. The post-PE syndrome: a new concept for chronic complications of pulmonary embolism. Blood Rev. 2014;28:221–6.

11. Frost A, Badesch D, Gibbs JSR, Gopalan D, Khanna D, Manes A, Oudiz R, Satoh T, Torres F, Torbicki A. Diagnosis of pulmonary hypertension. Eur Respir J. 2019;53:1801904.

12. Claeys M, Claessen G, La Gerche A, Petit T, Belge C, Meyns B, Bogaert J, Willems R, Claus P, Delcroix M. Impaired cardiac reserve and abnormal vascular load limit exercise capacity in chronic thromboembolic disease. JACC Cardiovasc Imaging. 2019;12:1444–56.

13. Axell RG, Messer SJ, White PA, McCabe C, Priest A, Statopoulou T, Drozdzynska M, Viscasillas J, Hinchy EC, Hampton-Till J, Alibhai HI, Morrell N, Pepke-Zaba J, Large SR, Hoole SP. Ventriculo-arterial coupling detects occult RV dysfunction in chronic thromboembolic pulmonary vascular disease. Physiol Rep. 2017;5(7):e13227.

14. McCabe C, White PA, Hoole SP, Axell RG, Priest AN, Gopalan D, Taboada D, Ross RM, Morrell NW, Shapiro LM, Pepke-Zaba J. Right ventricular dysfunction in chronic thromboembolic obstruction of the pulmonary artery: a pressure-volume study using the conductance catheter. J Appl Physiol. 2014;116:355–63.

15. van Kan C, van der Plas MN, Reesink HJ, van Steenwijk RP, Kloek JJ, Tepaske R, Bonta PI, Bresser P. Hemodynamic and ventilatory responses during exercise in chronic thromboembolic disease. J Thorac Cardiovasc Surg. 2016;152:763–71.

16. McCabe C, Deboeck G, Harvey I, Ross RM, Gopalan D, Screaton N, Pepke-Zaba J. Inefficient exercise gas exchange identifies pulmonary hypertension in chronic thromboembolic obstruction following pulmonary embolism. Thromb Res. 2013;132:659–65.

17. Guth S, Wiedenroth CB, Rieth A, Richter MJ, Gruenig E, Ghofrani HA, Arlt M, Liebetrau C, Prüfer D, Rolf A, Hamm CW, Mayer E. Exercise right heart catheterisation before and after pulmonary endarterectomy in patients with chronic thromboembolic disease. Eur Respir J. 2018;52:1800458.

18. McCabe C, Dimopoulos K, Pitcher A, Orchard E, Price LC, Kempny A, Wort SJ. Chronic thromboembolic disease following pulmonary embolism: time for a fresh look at old clot. Eur Respir J. 2020;55:1901934.

19. Dong C, Zhou M, Liu D, Long X, Guo T, Kong X. Diagnostic accuracy of computed tomography for chronic thromboembolic pulmonary hypertension: a systematic review and meta-analysis. PLoS One. 2015;10(4):e0126985.

20. Wang M, Wu D, Ma R, Zhang Z, Zhang H, Han K, Xiong C, Wang L, Fang W. Comparison of V/Q SPECT and CT angiography for the diagnosis of chronic thromboembolic pulmonary hypertension. Radiology. 2020;296:420–9.

21. Haramati A, Haramati LB. Imaging of chronic thromboembolic disease. Lung. 2020;198:245–55.

22. Shahin Y, Johns C, Karunasaagarar K, Kiely DG, Swift AJ. IodiNe subtraction mapping in the diagnosis of pulmonary chronIc thRomboEmbolic disease (INSPIRE): rationale and methodology of a cross-sectional observational diagnostic study. Contemp Clin Trials Commun. 2019;15:1004172.

23. Bunclark K, Newnham M, Chiu Y-D, Ruggiero A, Villar SS, Cannon JE, Coghlan G, Corris PA, Howard L, Jenkins D, Johnson M, Kiely DG, Ng C, Screaton N, Sheares K, Taboada D, Tsui S, Wort SJ, Pepke-Zaba J, Toshner M. A multicenter study of anticoagulation in operable chronic thromboembolic pulmonary hypertension. J Thromb Haemostasis. 2020;18:114–22.

24. Swietlik EM, Ruggiero A, Fletcher AJ, Taboada D, Knightbridge E, Harlow L, Harvey I, Screaton N, Cannon JE, Sheares KKK, Ng C, Jenkins DP, Pepke-Zaba J, Toshner MR. Eur Respir J. 2019;53:1801787. https://doi.org/10.1183/13993003.01787-2018.

25. Donahoe L, Vanderlaan R, Thenganatt J, McRae K, Bykova A, Moric J, Granton J, de Perrot M. Symptoms are more useful than echocardiography in patient selection for pulmonary endarterectomy. Ann Thorac Surg. 2017;104:1179–85.

26. Yıldızeli ŞO, Kepez A, Taş S, Yanartaş M, Durusoy AF, Erkılınç A, Mutlu B, Kaymaz C, Sunar H, Yıldızeli B. Pulmonary endarterectomy for patients with chronic thromboembolic disease. Anatol J Cardiol. 2018;19:273–8.

27. Taboada D, Pepke-Zaba J, Jenkins DP, Berman M, Treacy CM, Cannon JE, Toshner M, Dunning JJ, Ng C, Tsui SS, Sheares KK. Outcome of pulmonary endarterectomy in symptomatic chronic thromboembolic disease. Eur Respir J. 2014;44:1635–45.

28. Wiedenroth CB, Olsson KM, Guth S, Breithecker A, Haas M, Kamp JC, Fuge J, Hinrichs JB, Roller F, Hamm CW, Mayer E, Ghofrani HA, Meyer BC, Liebetrau C. Balloon pulmonary angioplasty for inoperable patients with chronic thromboembolic disease. Pulmonary Circ. 2018;8(1):1–6.

29. Inami T, Kataoka M, Kikuchi H, Goda A, Satoh T. Balloon pulmonary angioplasty for symptomatic chronic thromboembolic disease without pulmonary hypertension at rest. Int J Cardiol. 2019;289:116–8.

30. Coghlan JG. Balloon pulmonary angioplasty: does it have a role in CTED? Pulmonary Circ. 2018;8(1):2045893218754887.

Printed in the United States
by Baker & Taylor Publisher Services